HOUSE CALLS

*Memoirs of Life with a
Kentucky Doctor*

MEMORIAL EDITION

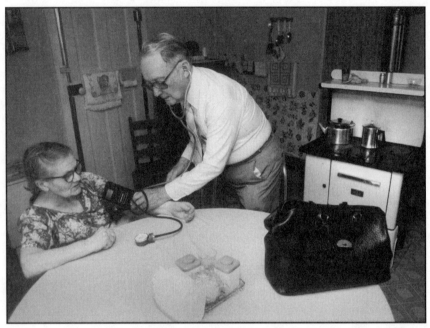

House call on Span Hill—Pearlie New.

HOUSE CALLS

Memoirs of Life with a Kentucky Doctor

MEMORIAL EDITION

by
Alma Dolen Roberts

Jesse Stuart Foundation
Ashland, Kentucky
2001

HOUSE CALLS

Memoirs of Life with a
Kentucky Doctor

Copyright © 2000 by Alma Dolen Roberts
Memorial Edition

Library of Congress Cataloging-in-Publication Data

Roberts, Alma Dolen, 1917-
   House calls : memoirs of life with a Kentucky doctor / by Alma Dolen Roberts.
   p. cm.
   ISBN 0-94-5084-85-4
   1. Roberts, Mack, 1903-2001 2. Physicians—Kentucky—Biography. 3. Medicine, Rural—Kentucky—History. I. Title

R154.R518 A3 2000
610'.92—dc21
[B]

Published by:
Jesse Stuart Foundation
P.O. Box 669 Ashland, Kentucky 41114
2001

Table of Contents

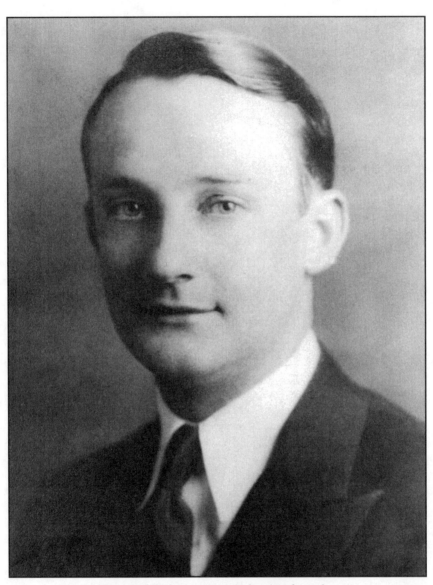

*Dr. Mack Roberts upon graduating from the
University of Loiusville Medical School in 1932.*

The physician's life "is compounded of the agony and glory, the weakness and the dread, the laughter and the drabness of humanity. About these things one cannot really afford to be merely clever. For in the final analysis we are all creatures laid low, at the mercy of physicians of nature and of God."

George N. Schuster

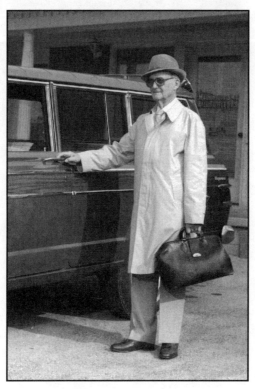

Going on a house call.

***This book is gratefully dedicated to
our dear family
and our faithful patients.***

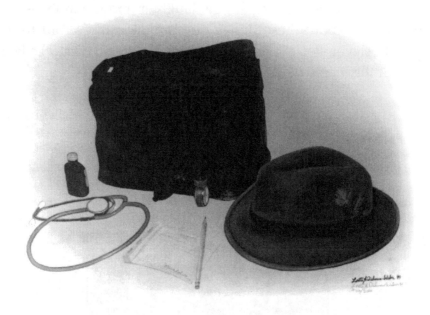

The Last House Call, tribute to Dr. Mack Roberts by Loretta A. Dishman-Webber, 1994

Introduction

For as much as many have taken in hand to set forth in order a declaration of those things which are most surely believed among us . . . It seemed good to me also, having had perfect understanding of all things from the very first, to write further of the things, wherein thou hast been instructed . . . .
(With apologies to the beloved physician, Luke)

Some few years ago I recorded many interesting occurrences that my husband, Dr. Mack Roberts, a physician, had experienced. Since that time Mack has been featured by many writers. WAVE television station of Louisville, Kentucky, filmed a documentary on him.

Others who have written knew the physician, but I, his wife, know both the physician and the man, as well as the milieu in which he lived.

If eight hundred books have been written about Napoleon, why can't mine be written about one who has devoted sixty-one years of his life (1932-1993) to practicing medicine in rural Kentucky at a time when stamina was as much needed as skill?

Many have requested I write such a book. "Give your rendition, tell your side of the story," they urged.

The ultimate justification for this attempt is that through this book future generations may learn that Mack Roberts was a man who served his time well. They will see a man of character and determination, a man of wit and fun, a dedicated doctor who loved his work, a man I think worthy of emulation. They may wish they could have shared his life. I only wish my ancestors had left their record for me.

Too, I hope this account will be read with profit and entertainment by those who have insisted on my writing it. I have tried to supply a fuller account than heretofore recorded and add to the portrait of this interesting man.

Writing this book has revealed many details of my husband's life I had not previously known, particularly those relating to his childhood. Now I know him better. Reliving our lives has been a joyful experience.

I have attempted to present this work chronologically. In Part I one will read of the doctor's birth, childhood, and education. In Part II I tell of *our* lives after I became his *wife* and *helper*.

In my story one will meet real-life, unforgettable characters (the names often fictitious). One will learn the joys and tribulations of a country doctor and his family.

This book is my own effort. I confess that I, a twelfth-hour writer, do not come to this project without certain biases and opinions. I state my own feelings. Just as the best prayers are from the heart, so, I think, is the best writing.

I feel a special debt of gratitude to Norma Cole, a dear friend—not for her assistance but for her encouragement. Indeed, she was my writing mentor. I also thank and appreciate the untiring effort of my new friend and typist, Sharon Robinson, and a dear family friend, Dr. Guy R. Woodall, for reading the manuscript and offering commentary.

PART I: 1903-1938
Birth, childhood, education
Health officer

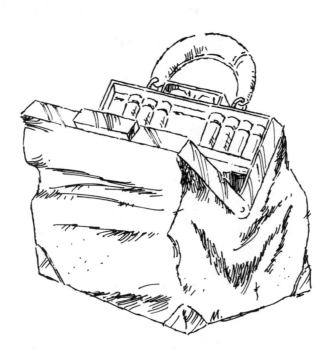

House Call

Dr. Mack Roberts remembers:

Rrringg, Rringg, Ring . . .

I get out of the bed and stumble into the hall to answer the phone.

"Hello."

"Hallo.

"Hello."

"Hallo, is this you, Doc?"

I can hardly hear the caller for the cacophony of the katy-dids outside our opened windows.

"This is Dr. Roberts," I answer.

"Doc, this is Jim Lee calling for Jake Brown. He says his wife's in labor and bad off. He needs you right away."

"Tell him to hurry," I hear Jake urge his neighbor.

I know Jake and his wife, Arzetta. I know where they live - quite a distance out in the country. I had delivered several children for them.

We had had a rain the night before. "Will I have any trouble getting there in my Jeep?" I ask. I knew the creek became the roadbed for a mile or so before I reached Jake's place.

"We're pretty shore you can make it 'cross the creek. Why, if you have any trouble, Dester, my boy, he will take you the rest of the way on a mule."

"I'll try it, but listen for me to blow my horn if my car drowns out. Tell Jake I'll be there."

I notice the absence of the clicking of telephone receivers on the party line; too late for eavesdroppers. The clock says 1:30 this mid-August morning.

I dress hurriedly. I put both medical bags into my vehicle and start on my twenty-mile trip.

My mind is on Jake Brown. Only a few days before, he had been in my office. He had complained of being unable to sleep. Not many men are afflicted with this problem. In my practice ninety percent of the insomniacs had been female victims, sometimes patients who had "cultivated their nerves," to use the terminology of an elderly spinster who scoffed at the idea of being unable to sleep. "I don't cultivate my nerves," she had bragged.

A typical mountain man, Jake lived in the southern part of the county, up a hollow in a weathered cabin with a lean-to kitchen. A day laborer, he probably earned $1 a day plus his noon meal, working for neighboring farmers. Sometimes he worked in the log woods cutting timber. Fiftyish, he was of average height, sturdy and slightly stooped.

That day in the absence of a button for one of the galluses on his faded Duck Head bibbed overalls, Jake had substituted a Kentucky button (a ten-penny nail). His greasy flop brim hat had been worn so long it resembled him.

Had he been so strapped financially that the upcoming doctor bill for delivering the baby kept him awake?

A fox dashes across the road and brings me back to the present. The rough graveled road is full of mud holes deep enough to drown a young'un. President F.D. Roosevelt's WPA workers had improved many of our roads, but they had not gotten to this one.

The new moon, looking like a trimmed fingernail, hangs in the southwestern sky. Heat lightning plays across the western horizon. The day had been a scorcher.

Bugs spat my windshield and find their way into the open Jeep. The night air smells of new-mown hay and the scent of dusty roads. The katydids are earsplitting out here in this wooded countryside. Houses are in darkness. Tired farmers are enjoying their deserved rest. I must be the sole person out tonight.

In my musing I remember Jake had said "Hurry." Rough roads notwithstanding, I step on the gas and bound along at twenty-five miles per hour.

It strikes me that Jake has a houseful of children; chances are my patient won't dally around with this delivery.

I hope Jake in his excitement doesn't have his neighbor phone and wake my wife again before I can get there; that often happens.

Was it last winter? It must have been the winter before that I had delivered the last baby for them. That had been a memorable case—unforgettable. That night had certainly been a contrast to this night weatherwise.

Snow had triple blanketed the earth. The temperature had been in single digits. I hadn't yet bought my four-wheel drive Jeep. We had two family cars, one of which I had bought second hand during W.W.II. We called it "Mousie" because we had discovered a mouse in it.

For my trip to Jake's I had checked both cars for gas. I thought Mousie had enough fuel for the trip.

I had put chains on the hind wheels, donned my long johns and dressed in my heaviest clothing including my Mackinaw coat. I yanked on my four buckle overshoes, picked up my wool gloves and cap that had ear flaps. I started for Jake's.

I had crept along, sometimes slipping and sliding, tire chains clanking. I dared not touch my brakes. I got stuck once. A kind neighbor pulled me out of the ditch with a mule. Snow crunched under our footsteps. On the final miles of the trip I had become a trailblazer. The road was not as hazardous where there had been no traffic.

When I arrived at Jake's, he was in a terribly nervous state. There had, of course, been a long wait for my arrival. The baby had not been born. Babies did sometimes arrive first.

The details of that delivery may have faded but I remember two. Hot water had been ready for me, but the room was frigid. I quickly sterilized all necessary instruments and gloves and started to examine Arzetta. She wore long underwear. "Aren't you going to put on a gown?" I asked.

"Naw," she said. "There's a hole in my underwear down there."

I understood Arzetta's reasoning. I recalled a former patient whose feet were frostbitten during prolonged labor in a room no colder than this. She had big black blisters on both feet 2 or 2 1/2 inches in diameter.

Arzetta would not be wearing long underwear tonight!

After that baby had been born, I had asked the necessary information for the birth certificate. "Number in order of birth" the form requested.

"How many children do you already have?" I asked, with pen poised.

Jake looked at his wife. "Count 'em."

"You count 'em," she said.

Silence.

It occurred to me that it was considered bad luck to count one's children. I waited.

"Nine," Arzetta blurted out.

"A fine family. How are they divided, Jake?"

"Half and half," he said, beaming.

How did they feed that many?

Now I'm at the creek. I halt to inspect it. It is plenty full. Can I make it or will I have to wade over? I don't have time to spend in contemplation. I enter the stream cautiously. I am familiar with the course to take. Keep near the left bank for a mile, then veer to the right and abruptly to the right to avoid a drop off.

I move carefully along splashing water. Perhaps the water will wash the mud off my vehicle. I think I've about made it when my engine sputters and conks out. I'm in deep water!

I can wade out, but I don't want to leave my car in the creek. What if we get a big rain? It could wash my Jeep away. My two bags would be heavy to carry the mile to Jake's house.

What can I do? Jake will be in a tizzy. Thank goodness, his wife is much calmer. Typical of women, they are more patient and endure pain better than men.

I wait a few minutes, I notice my gas supply is low. With the engine in gear, I step on the starter. Luckily, the car lurches forward. The starter had propelled me just far enough to get into shallower water.

Again, I wait a few minutes for my engine to dry. I step on the starter. The engine sputters, coughs and spits, then pulls the car out of the water. That was close.

What will I do if I get stranded out here? That lightning I'd seen—but heat lightning isn't ominous, is it? I could always walk out, by Tick Ridge. I had done plenty of walking and riding mules or horses before I had bought my Jeep.

I hurry on up the road alongside the creek and finally by the light of my car see the bulk of Jake standing by the road. He waves me up the lane and into his yard.

"Hurry, Doc, hurry."

I get out of the car and hand him the O.B. (obstetrics) bag. I carry the other bag. The air is warm, oppressive. Somewhere a cat squalls. An owl hoots mournfully.

"The baby hasn't arrived yet?" I say.

"No, no, Doc. Hurry!" Jake kicks at a menacing dog.

I trail Jake through the weedy yard toward the house. Where is the light? We enter a room lighted by a globeless lantern that gives off more smell than light. I almost collide with a woman who carries a tea kettle spouting steam.

"We don't have much light," Jake apologizes.

The lantern simply made the darkness visible.

I am stunned. What a challenge! I hotfoot it to my car, turn it and aim the bright headlights directly into the house. I leave the motor running to keep my battery from going dead. How long will my gas last?

I quickly sterilize gloves and instruments and check Arzetta. It won't be long until she delivers. Her pains are getting closer and severe. She has a gown on this time.

I'm thankful I got across the stream or Jake would have been in worse condition than his wife who moans intermittently with each pang of pain.

I sit on a chair that has a board across the frame. I worry about my gas supply.

I discover the house is full of locusts. That seventeen-year cycle had rolled around again. I had heard their "Phara-o-ro-roah, Pharoo-oo-oh" the last few days. I also hear subdued twittering in the kitchen, the older children probably. The young ones are usually farmed out among the kinfolk at such a time.

Jake and I make small talk. I learn that Arzetta has worked in the garden that day. Jake is antsy, constantly going in and out of the house.

I keep my eyes on Arzetta and my ears on my car engine, to know that my gas supply has not dwindled out.

The flickering, smoking lantern sputters. Insects are attracted to it. (The house has no screens.) They flutter in too close and "zap"–one is cremated.

I remember another case where I was left in total darkness with my crying, expectant mother while her husband carried the lantern, their only source of light, with him to the spring to get water. That lantern had had a smoky globe.

My patient's pains become harder and closer together. I put a few drops of chloroform on a piece of gauze and drop it into a glass for her to smell, to ease the pain. Jake mops his sweaty brow with a blue bandanna and walks the floor.

The baby arrives, kicking and squalling. No need to spank this one. His arrival makes three people happy—his mother, his father, and me.

After tying and severing the umbilical cord, I put drops of silver nitrate in the infant's eyes, a requirement to prevent gonorrheal infection of the eyes.

I weigh the little fellow—8 lbs., 14 oz. I turn him over to the awaiting neighbor. She cleans him with melted lard (they had no baby oil), dresses him in a shirt and diaper and lays him beside his mother.

Jake steps around briskly. "He's a fine one, ain't he, Doc?"

"Looks like a prize fighter," I say. Inasmuch as I can see in the glaring light and shadows, he has all ten fingers and toes.

Arzetta is fine. Though she has had no prenatal care, so far, she has experienced no difficulty in childbearing.

"You're soon going to have all the workhands you can use, Jake."

"They'll come in handy."

"What are you going to name him?"

"Otto," the parents answer simultaneously.

Sounds from the kitchen are louder—giggling and talking.

While I fill out the birth certificate, Arzetta cuddles the baby. Jake is bent over them.

What a welcome! You would think the newborn was their firstborn.

I check mother and baby once more and pack my bags to leave.

Jake digs into the watch pocket of his overalls and pulls out a wad of $1 bills and hands them to me. I don't count them. Knowing Jake, there are twenty-five of them as twenty-five dollars is the going charge for a delivery. He and Arzetta appear to be very appreciative of my help.

Jake and I pick up my bags, and he accompanies me to the car.

The air is cooler and the cicadas are quiet. The moon has emerged from a cloud cover. Jake's dog that had growled when I arrived wags his tail and pads beside me. I hear a nearby mockingbird showing off, putting on his predawn show.

"I shore am glad you come," Jake said. "Much obliged, Doc." He heads back for the house.

I turn my Jeep and check my gas gauge. I think I have enough fuel to get home.

Now to get back across the stream. I approach it warily. No problem this time. I'm out!

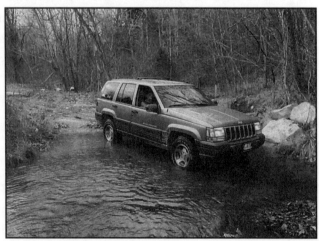

House call—a common occurrence.

I feel good. I have again witnessed the miracle of birth. Jake's and Arzetta's baby is fortunate to have such wonderful parents, I say to myself. Though the room for the infant in the house might be limited, there is plenty of love for him in his parents' hearts; that is what counts.

Farmers are still asleep. The whole world seems asleep— everything except the bugs. They still "spat" my windshield. I'm tired and ready for sleep. A creature, perhaps a groundhog, starts to cross in front of me, thinks better of it and backs off.

Home at last, I pull into my driveway. I'm blocked by a clay-spattered trap of a truck. I stop.

A husky, grinning, bearded fellow gets out of the car and approaches. I recognize him. He is from Bugwood, twelve miles out of town. I know he has come for me. His wife is overdue.

First I must fill my gas tank at that 24-hour service station on the south end of town.

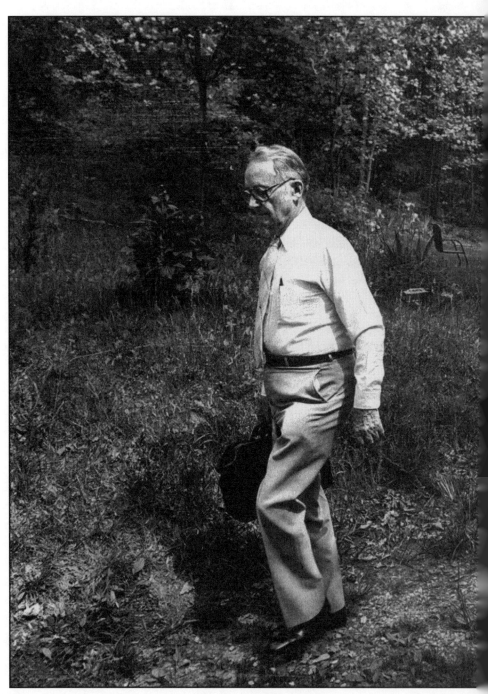

House call on Elk Ridge, 1987.

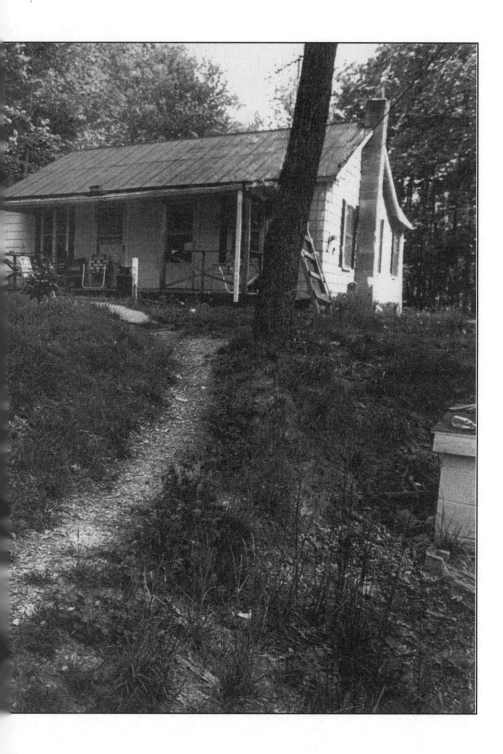

Birth

In the third year of the twentieth century, the Wright brothers made their first flight. It lasted twelve seconds. President Theodore Roosevelt sent a message around the world by Marconi's wireless in twelve minutes. It did not announce the birth of a ten-pound son to Rhodes Rankin Roberts and Verona Clementine Vickery Roberts at Cooper in Wayne County, Kentucky, July 24, 1903.

The parents brought the baby to the home of his paternal grandparents at Oil Valley—not from the hospital, but from the residence of the maternal grandparents, Irvin and Mary Thornton Vickery.

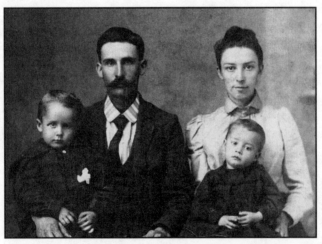

*Dr. Roberts' parents, Rhodes and Rona Roberts
and brothers, Hobart and Ottis.*

Because of the illness of her father, the expectant mother had been called to her parents' home. While the mother visited with her parents, Irvin and Mary Thornton Vickery, the baby chose, as babies usually do, the inopportune time to be born.

Dr. C. B. Rankin rode his horse the seven miles from Monticello to Cooper to deliver the child, who would later become his colleague.

Room was available for the newborn baby at the home of the paternal grandparents, Andrew Jackson Roberts and Susan Clark Roberts. In fact, his parents lived with the grandparents along with sons Hobart and Ottis.

The comfortable, two-story brick house with a dogtrot had been built in 1837. The Rhodes Roberts family lived in an upstairs bedroom.

Jackson Roberts had moved to Oil Valley from Kidd's Crossing in Wayne County in 1897. He and his oldest son, Bolen, had purchased a large farm from Mr. Sammy Ingram.

The parents named the baby "Roy." At that time, an Irishman by the name of McElroy supervised the building of the Oil Valley turnpike in Wayne County. In playing with the baby, someone called him McElroy. Later, the name was shortened to "Mack." The nickname stuck.

In this patriarchal society, the child grew and was loved greatly by parents, brothers, grandparents and four unmarried aunts who still lived at home.

The little boy wore dresses, as was the custom of the period. He had long blond curls. The father wanted his son to look like a boy, and he had his curls shorn. That act brought the adoring aunts to tears.

Little Mack lost the distinction of being "the baby" when Harry soon joined the family, bringing the number of sons to four.

In another year or so, Harry lost the special attention when displaced by Kermit. Now there were five children plus the parents sharing the homestead with grandparents and aunts.

What a change this must have been for Verona, the boys' mother. "Miss Ronie," as she was called before and after marriage, had been a school teacher. She had attended the Doublehead Academy in Hall Valley, where she prepared for the teacher's examination.

She had taught school at Gophertown, near Mt. Pisgah, before the turn of the century for the enviable salary of twenty dollars per month. Room and board cost ten dollars. She taught at Backbone, near Cabell, and at Sumpter. She then acquired a teaching position at Burfield—just across the hill from the Roberts place.

The gallant, black-mustached Rhodes Roberts soon discovered the pretty brown-eyed Vickery girl known for her intellect.

Their friendship flowered into a romance that was followed by marriage in 1897. Rhodes took his bride to his father's home.

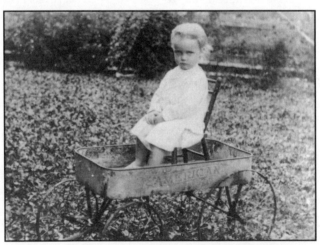

Mack in a dress and long blond curls.

Milestones

When we left the "gay nineties" and entered into the twentieth century, America was the world's greatest industrial power, but sixty percent of all Americans still lived in rural communities. The largest occupation was farming. We had half the world's railroad mileage, pumped half its oil and mined a third of its steel and gold.

We had a total of forty-five states.

Many families were almost self-sufficient. One person out of two belonged to a church. Love still expressed itself in a kiss with marriage as the almost inevitable consequence. Right was right; wrong was wrong. Infidelity was not condoned. Almost nobody got a divorce.

Woman's place was in the home, tending the children. She did not have the right to vote. However, early in the century women began to try to change this concept of their role in society. The National American Woman's Suffrage Association became more active. Women's colleges began to send out alumnae.

Teddy Roosevelt wielded the big stick and projected our might abroad.

In 1906 our 46th state, Oklahoma, was added to the Union.

The Model T had not yet replaced the horsedrawn carriage.

Telephones brought about instant communication.

Sears Roebuck and Co. and Montgomery Ward brought shopping to the home.

Patent medicine vied with home remedies.

Modern sports took off during these years: football's Rose Bowl, tennis' Davis Cup, baseball's World Series, and the first Olympic Games in America.

Silent movies made their debut, and Hollywood enticed.

The new music was ragtime.

Public libraries appeared. Magazines such as *The Atlantic Monthly* and *Colliers* were welcomed. The *Saturday Evening Post* and *Ladies Home Journal* made their appearance.

Progress notwithstanding, the Roberts family lived more in accord with the nineteenth century. It would be some time before their work became mechanized. Old ways persisted. Foremost was the rearing of the children. Otherwise, their lives revolved around church, school and simple pleasures. Theirs was a gradual involvement in the revolution that altered the American home.

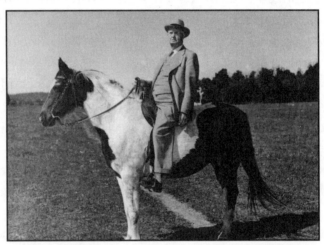

Dr. C.B. Rankin, a dear friend, who delivered Mack (1903) and who later became his colleague.

Oil on Troubled Water

These were not the best of times for grandfather Andrew Jackson Roberts. He lived in fear of losing his farm. At a propitious time, around 1900 a pioneer oil company struck oil on the Jackson and Bolen Roberts farms. The financial tide began to turn. Pennsylvanians flocked to Wayne County in search of the liquid gold.

But disaster struck when Jackson's son Hayes, age thirty and Jackson's unmarried daughter Ethel, age twenty-four, both died of tuberculosis. The discovery of oil on the Roberts' property probably proved to be a curse rather than a godsend. It is remembered that among the oil workers who lived and boarded at the Roberts home was a man who had a dreadful, incessant cough. The family believed that it was from him that Hayes and Ethel contracted the fatal disease. Mack's Grandmother Susan Clark Roberts died two years later of an undiagnosed illness.

Two years after his wife died, "Uncle Jackson," as he was called by the neighbors, acclaimed as quite a character, shaved his whiskers and began to "look over" the ladies. Tipped off by a friend, he sojourned to Rock Creek in the eastern part of the county, to meet one fine, energetic lady many years his junior. Jackson liked what he found.

Florence Phipps Dolen was George Dolen's widow. "Miss Florence" and Jackson did not tarry long until they were married. She would bring two unmarried daughters to the Roberts household.

This brought about a reappraisal of housing.

Though two of Jackson's daughters had married by this time and another, Aunt Lytha, had left for Valparaiso, Indiana, to attend school, the house bulged with two families. The Rhodes Roberts family numbered seven; togetherness reigned.

Money from his oil field enabled Uncle Bolen to purchase a farm at Mill Springs, and he, in turn, sold his part of the Ingram farm to his father, Andrew Jackson Roberts.

Uncle Bolen retained the oil rights on the farm he sold. (A well on the property is still in production.)

Since Rhodes had managed his father's farm for a number of years (and continued to do so until his father's death), his father gave him the B.E. Roberts farm. (The father was well into his seventies at this time.) The Bolen Roberts farm consisted of one hundred acres of cleared ground and two hundred acres of woodland.

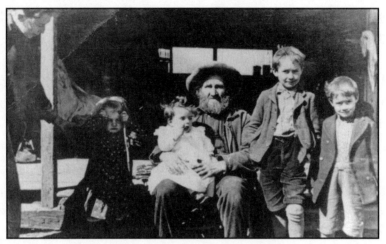

(left to right) Extreme left, Mack's Mother, Mack pouting, Harry in Grandfather Jackson's lap, Hobart and Ottis.

"We still lived with our grandfather," Mack said, "when he brought his Christmas bride, twenty-five years younger than he, to the Oil Valley home.

"Hobart, Ottis and I must have given her a royal welcome. We had just skinned a polecat, and of course, we came inside to warm."

Miss Florence's two daughters, Ola Dolen (Hucaby) and Temple Dolen (Cox) would join the family a couple of months later.

"There was always harmony in the family circle," Mack said.

March 7, 1910, Rhodes pulled up stakes and moved his family into the log house on his own farm, recently vacated by his brother, Bolen. Mack was six years old, and he still remembers the date!

The New House

The setting sun is reflected from the windows of the almshouse as brightly as from the rich man's abode; the snow melts before his door as early in the spring.

Henry David Thoreau

The Robertses' three-room log house made of rough hewn poplar logs sat on a hillside at the head of a valley surrounded by wooded hills full of varmints.

There was no yard, just a ragged sweep of grass and weeds down to a branch and a two-rut, jolt-wagon road that dead-ended at the Roberts place. A wood-burning fireplace dominated the family room called "the big house."

Here, in the new home, the children would be isolated from other children, except perhaps on weekends. It could be considered a desolate place in which to live. Nevertheless, the boys knew nothing of loneliness.

Though the horizon was near, no getting away from it, their playground reached as far as the eye could see, and all that they saw they owned.

The brothers were no more alone than the frogs in the branch nor the birds in the treetops.

Uninhibited by parental discipline, except for misbehavior, the boys were born free—to romp and roam as they wished. They scattered like baby quail.

In the new home, the three older boys—Hobart, Ottis and

Mack–slept in the unheated loft, reached through darkness at night by a ladder. The wailing March wind, whipping through branches, sounded lonesome. Trees creaked and popped. Bare apple tree limbs lashed the one window in the attic, but the trio snuggled into their buoyant homemade featherbeds. Dressed in long underwear they were warm under six or eight quilts made by their mother.

In bed, Mack liked to listen to the sounds of the night: the roar of the March wind, the baying of foxhounds, the "whoo-whoo" of a nearby owl, the "thump" in the downstairs fireplace when a chunk of wood burned through and crashed onto the hearth.

The young fellow recognized the tinkle of an icicle when touched by a bough or something. Sounds from the barn were easily interpreted: the plaintive bawl of a calf separated from its mother, the mother's long, drawn-out "moo-oo-oo," and a rebel mule kicking a stall. The house shuddered and creaked.

How comforting it was to hear the murmur of his parents downstairs, talking over the day's events. But sleep crept on.

Early in the dead silence of the morning, he is awakened by the exuberant crowing of a rooster. The contest is on. The Robertses' Dominique roosters compete with the neighbor's Wyandottes as far as a mile away—until dawn.

Often the children wake to find frost on the quilts from their breath. Sometimes when they jump out of bed they track in bare feet through snow that has sifted in through cracks around the frost-etched window. (In April, apple blossoms blew in through the same openings.)

The little boys rise early, when called, along with the household. They descend the ladder and dress in front of the roaring fire in the big house. In the lamp-lighted kitchen they hear their mother grinding coffee beans with a hand coffee mill.

They gather milk pails from nails on the kitchen wall and follow their father to the barn to help milk and feed the stock before breakfast.

"My father said I could milk when I was so little I had to stand and reach up to the teats," Mack says.

The glacial air cuts through the lads like a scalpel. Undaunted, they try to outrun the wind. If it is snowing, they might try to catch snowflakes on their tongues. They are followed by dogs, Duke, a white dog, and Shep, a little black dog.

At the barn the boys are greeted by fattening hogs who grunt and squeal for corn, horses who whinny for corn and hay, and cows who "moo" for nubbins. "Why should they eat before we do?" somebody asks.

Even in cold weather the barn smells of manure, animals, milk, hay and leather.

With chores finished, the brothers start to the house. They stop at the watering trough where the water is piped from the spring to the livestock. They wash their faces and hands under the spout. The icy water makes their faces tingle and oftentimes freezes in their hair as they race, blowing on their knuckles, back toward the house. White smoke curls from the chimney.

The cold air whips into the house with them. The boys push and scuffle to get close to the open fire, almost upsetting the churn on the hearth. They stand with back to fire, hands behind them. Steam rises from their damp, cold clothing.

The aroma of coffee brewing in the blue-speckled granite coffeepot fills the room. Mack tasted coffee once. He didn't like it; he never tasted it again.

Bacon sizzles in a cast-iron skillet. The black teakettle sends up puffs of vapor. The father has built the fire in the wood cookstove by carrying a shovelful of live coals from the fireplace.

Their mother stokes the cookstove with cobs and wood. Her dark hair is coiled in a tidy knot atop her head. She wears a multipurpose apron; her sleeves are rolled. She has flour on her hands from biscuit-making in a wooden tray. The baby is still asleep in bed.

"Breakfast is ready," she announces. Her children are ready, too. They eat by the faint light of a kerosene lamp. Bacon or sausage from their own hogs; butter, sorghum or homemade jellies are staples. From time to time they have hot mush. Fried salmon cakes are a real treat.

Rice and oatmeal, creamy and chewy (not the instant kind), are winter breakfast foods, as are fried Irish and sweet potatoes. Sweet potatoes glisten with sugar sprinkled on top of the slices.

Not many eggs were used during the winter months; they were scarce and valuable. They were exchanged for other foods at the country store. Not until eggs were as cheap as ten cents a dozen were they consumed in quantity. Goose eggs, kept in an open-top bushel gourd, brought five cents each.

Sometimes when the boys found frozen eggs, they roasted them in hot ashes in the fireplace. They roasted potatoes in the same way.

The children learn the work ethic at an early age from both parents by precept and example. On their first winter in the log house, the three oldest boys, six, nine and eleven, are assigned the task of providing wood for the demanding fireplace and cookstove.

On a cold frosty morning, with a crosscut saw, they fell a tree and lop off its branches with an ax. With their yoke of steers, Buck and Dick, and guided from the left by a line, they snake the log to the woodlot. They saw it into appropriate sizes for the fireplace and cookstove. This daily task consumes most of a short winter day.

The great outdoors serves as laboratory—their science, zoology and botany books. They learn by observation. They witness birth and death among the barnyard animals.

Winter nights are the most fun. On those evenings the boys go hunting, except for Sunday nights. "Mama forbade hunting on Sunday nights," Mack said.

Three mittened fellows, warmly dressed, are about to disturb the balance of nature in search of their fortune.

It is the dead of winter; the wind is raw. The boys light their lantern and follow the yelps of Duke and Shep. They are accompanied by their guardian angels.

Ottis, who is short of stature, bump-bumps the lantern along against every obstacle a foot off the ground. He follows the leader of most of their childhood expeditions, Hobart, who carries the rifle and hunting knife. Mack trails. They walk from one puddle of light to another.

The brothers crawl on all fours under a rusted barbed wire fence and tread their own familiar path into the dark and forbidding forest. The wind rattles bare branches; pines sough overhead. They smell like Christmas. Stars twinkle in the sky.

The siblings push and pull the lagging one up precipitous moss-covered rocks. They scoot down the other side of the boulder. They are alert to all the sounds of the woods: a hunter's horn, the bark of a fox, the crash of a dead limb.

The youngsters descend into a ravine. They cling to bushes and sometimes go head-over-heels into the hollow.

"We could tell when Shep and Duke had treed, by their barks," Mack says.

When one of the boys shoots by lantern light at a coon, down it falls. The dogs pounce on it—but are driven away. Animals were often skinned where killed and the pelt carried home.

If they didn't have their gun with them, they shook a possum out of a sapling and let the dogs get it for them.

"Look, how fat that possum is. He's been eating 'simmons."

The boys journey on, treading lightly. "Wait for me; a briar snatched my cap."

Something makes a grunting sound. "What was that?" the wary kids wonder.

"Once in a while we'd hear a wildcat squall—away back in the mountains," Mack says. "That quickened our step and sent cold chills up our backs!"

Another hair-raising noise was the eerie call of a screech owl, or was it a panther?

One moonlit night they heard the sound like a woman screaming. "It's a panther!" one yelled. The boys beat their shadows home by ten lengths. "Shep and Duke bolted for home with us."

They set traps and baited them with meat skins.

Early in the silent, frosty morning, bundled in so many clothes they can hardly walk, they plod through mud or snowdrift for a daily check on traps. Overshoes were unheard of. They learned to waterproof their shoes by rubbing them with tallow.

The morning sounds are muted, no barking dogs or quacking ducks. Crows wing their way westward.

The boys' breaths are like steam from a teakettle; their cheeks are red and chapped.

Mission accomplished, they return with prize or disappointment. If they have made a catch, they have an extra spring to their step.

"Once we caught a weasel," Mack says. "That was the stinkiest thing I ever smelled."

Weasels were the culprits that invaded the chicken houses and killed their chickens. They left the chickens lying dead after sucking out their blood.

Many of those boy excursions were followed by a spell of the croup. This did not deter the hardy trappers.

Animals caught were killed, skinned, and the hides nailed to boards to dry.

Mack says, "A fur buyer came around every two or three weeks for our pelts. Gray fox pelts sold for $2.50 each. A red fox pelt brought five dollars. Coon hides brought five to six dollars. A black polecat pelt brought three dollars. A possum hide brought from fifty cents to a dollar fifty, according to size."

Their dogged pursuit of varmints earned them Christmas spending money. With the money they bought candy, bananas and oranges. Bananas and oranges were available only during cold weather because of lack of refrigeration in shipping.

Once the boys spent some of their money for a 'smoke gun.' "We ordered it and used it to puff smoke into animal dens to rout the creature. We didn't want our friends to know we had this 'secret weapon,' so we carried it in a sack.

"At 10:00 one night we got Uncle George Orr out of bed," Mack says, "to help us get a coon out of a tree.

"One day as we made our rounds to check our traps, we met a neighbor—an oil worker. He carried a steel trap—one of ours. 'Here boys, I hooked your trap,' he said. He handed it to us with little apparent embarrassment."

Work on the farm by the children went unpaid, moneywise; allowances were unheard of. Farm children were the ones to whom little is given and of whom much is required. Weren't they fed, clothed and housed, just as the work animals were fed and housed? They earned their keep.

In the early part of the twentieth century there were no paper routes for earning money, at least in the country; no "carry out" grocerybag jobs, or work at fast-food eating places. The boys no more had a lawn mower than the modern child has a yoke of steers.

Hunting and trapping provided the means to get money to spend for their own wants. They also earned money in the summertime by picking blackberries for ten cents a gallon.

When the boys grew older and weren't busy at assigned tasks, such as sledding fodder to the cattle, they hunted squirrels or rabbits. They became excellent marksmen. Mack, though right-handed, shoots left-handed. I've never known him to miss a target even into his 90's.

Black Gold

The discovery of oil on the Jackson Roberts place had put money into their coffers. Part of each monthly oil check had been brought home in gold, placed in a cigar box, and kept in the closet. The new industry also changed an isolated way of living into one that hummed with people and activity.

Though the trailblazers had arrived earlier, others continued to follow. They arrived at the Ramsey Hotel in Monticello, Kentucky, by stage coach. They were a breed distinct, a rugged band of lease grabbers, speculators, rig workers—all "wildcatting."

The newcomers dressed in khaki riding breeches and flannel shirts. They wore high-top laced leather boots with a red sock cuff. They had names uncommon to the natives: Orr, André, Geiger, Cafferty, Motter, Geason, Slobam, Burwahl. Many were of German descent. They brought new customs to the rural community. A number of them boarded at the Jackson Robertses, taking two of his daughters for their wives.

The dirt road past the Rhodes Roberts home became a thoroughfare to the Still House oil field. Workers passed daily hauling supplies.

Right below the home, wells on the B. E. Roberts lease were in full production. In fact, the first well drilled in the area is where Rhodes later built his home. That well # 1 produced 250 barrels daily for several days until put on a pump.

Originally the lease owner's royalty was one-tenth of the oil check. Later, he received one-eighth. One lease owner objected strenuously to the latter ruling. "I want one-tenth," he argued.

"Locations," probable sites for wells, were three hundred feet apart.

"Uncle Bolen had a dozen or so wells pumping at the same time," Mack says.

The "thump, thump" of the drilling machine, the clatter of tools, the hiss of the steam boiler, and the shouting of men delivering wood echoed throughout the hills and hollows. The smell of gas and the sound of "barkers" from the engines pumping oil were hardly noticed.

Today Mack points out many sites of wells. "That was # 21 out there on the bench," a terrace or shelf midway up the hill, out from the old home. "It was one of the later ones to 'go out'" (become unprofitable). He speaks in the vernacular of the petroleum industry. "Such wells were 'plugged' to keep water from seeping into the oil pool."

Oil was found on the Abijah Burnett place just up the hill from the Roberts farm. Mack says, "A father and son owned some wells on that property. They came out from Monticello every few days, a distance of eight or nine miles, to oversee the work on the lease; they barely eked out a living.

"They shared one bicycle. The father rode a mile or so, parked the bike by the fence and walked on. The son who had walked during this time, came along, got on the bicycle and rode his mile or so."

The two had set their Standard rig and had their wood hauled in, ready to drill another well. New Domain Oil Company came in and bought their lease. The new owners proceeded to drill the well. They got a "good well."

Such was the luck of the industry.

Mack tells of seeing a Star Drilling machine moved by horse-power up a mountain. "They had twenty-six mules hitched to the rig. Of course, not all of the mules pulled at the same time," he adds.

The Roberts children were well schooled in the oil business. They even witnessed the "shooting" of a well with nitroglycerine—to make the well more productive.

Other than the very early years when the aunts were still at home, the boys spent their early years mainly in an adult male society.

Childhood

What are little boys made of, made of?
What are little boys made of?
Frogs and snails and puppy-dog tails
That's what little boys are made of.

At the first hint of dawn, the Kentucky cardinals sound a wake-up call for our young naturalists—for another day of adventure: chasing butterflies, searching for the lucky four-leaf clover, sucking the nectar from the fragrant honeysuckle, searching for hens' nests in the tickly straw in the hay loft, trapping a bumblebee in a flower and listening to it fuss. They might flush a covey of quail, or rock a hornet's nest and then run for their lives. They liked to initiate a conversation with a bobwhite by imitating its call.

Like every other child in the neighborhood, they frolicked among the lightning bugs at dusk and collected them in a jar; or they caught crawdads by hand in the branch, then turned them loose.

The naughty kids tied a string to a jar fly's leg, and held the string while the insect buzzed around their heads.

On a scorching hot summer day, the little Roberts rascals might trap a horsefly, stick a chicken feather in its tail, and watch it zigzag across a field white with daisies.

The not-so-angelic fellows were guilty of tying a string to a grain of corn, feeding it to a chicken, then withdrawing string, corn intact!

After supper, they hear the frogs in the branch. "Knee deep, knee deep," call the little frogs.

"You'll drown; you'll drown," answers papa bullfrog.

In April "the voice of the turtle dove is heard in the land." At dusk the whippoorwill gives its frantic call. Wildflowers seem to spring up overnight.

The Roberts rovers knew where the sweet williams grew; where to find the jack-in-the-pulpit, columbine, bloodroot and an anemone they called the "whippoorwill plant." Their mother received many bouquets from tightly clenched fists.

Though young, the children had an appreciation of beauty.

Occasionally the trio stopped dead in their tracks and listened to the two short blasts of the Rowena Steamboat that plied the Cumberland River. The noise signaled the boat would stop at Norman's Landing. The air had to be calm for the sound to reach them, a distance of fifteen miles as the crow flies.

The boys were familiar with the Bassett Sawmill whistle in Monticello.

Not only did the surrounding hills and hollows abound with wild animals, birds and flowers, there were chiggers, ticks, and poison ivy. Rattlesnakes and copperheads were plentiful. Although the father suffered a copperhead bite, the children escaped.

"We liked to clean out the branch in the spring," Mack said. "We'd burn the dead grass and canes. The canes, when burned, popped like firecrackers."

Mack tells of his first time to shoot a shotgun.

"We had been losing our baby chicks to hawks. Every afternoon about the same time a hawk circled around, swooped down and carried off a 'diddle.'

"One afternoon when the hawk made its appearance, I went for my .22 rifle.

"'Take the shotgun,' my mother advised."

Mack was only seven or eight years old and had never used a shotgun.

"I laid my 20 gauge, single barrel shotgun across the top of a pole bean teepee, and let him have it.

"The sound reverberated throughout the hollow.

"I found the baby chick inside the garden fence, dead. I figured the hawk had escaped, but I found it on the other side of the fence, dead also."

And so the kids romped through summer.

These were the best of times.

Peddlers

"Mama, Mama," the Roberts kids call as they race down the lane to meet a short fellow humped under a backpack. "The peddler is comin'..."

Peddlers came, on foot, three or four times a year. They traveled all over the country, they even found customers in the remotest hideaways. Peddlers usually spent the night at the same patron's home each trip.

Mack says, "The peddlers were from Russia, supposedly. They pronounced it Roosha. They had queer names. One packman, named Site Olive, always stayed at Mr. Will Elam's."

Another peddler, a crippled man with both legs off below his knees, came on crutches. He took short cuts across the fields, climbed rail fences, rocked through mud holes, but he called on his customers.

Mack says, "We could hardly wait for the peddler to let his big, leather bag thump on the floor, then display his colorful trifles and trinkets. I remember among other goods he had kitchen gadgets, shoe buttoners, gold beads, coloring books, crayons, storybooks, laces, and spectacles.

"Many people, whose eyesight had failed, counted on the peddler to take care of their optical needs. The elderly tried on pair after pair of "specs" with narrow lenses, until they found a pair that would allow them to see a picture on the wall—then bought the glasses."

Peddlers no longer came after World War I.

Creativity

Creativity ran wild with the Roberts brothers. They made their own baseball by unraveling an old wool sock and rewinding the yarn on a small sponge rubber ball.

They devised a popgun from a joint of cane: a stick plunger dislodged thunderwood berries or a chewed-up paper wad—causing a loud "pop." They learned that teachers were not fond of popguns.

Similarly, they contrived a squirt gun using a pith-free joint of elder. With a plunger they suctioned water from a container and squirted someone.

The brothers made their own bows and arrows. Mack says, "Sometimes Pap (Grandfather Jackson) whittled us a bow of cedar." They had a quiver of sourwood switches.

To make a spear for their arrow, they drove a small nail into an empty .38 shell and slipped it onto the end of the arrow. Ottis accidentally speared a cow with such a weapon.

The boys made their own wagons. They searched until they found a blackgum pole about a foot in diameter. From the pole they cut four two-inch sections for the wheels. They bored through the center of each section and put them on front and back axles. They nailed boards from front to back.

In much the same way they made sleds.

The children lay on their stomachs on the sleds and careened wildly down steep hillsides.

The boys walked tall on homemade stilts; they made their own slingshots. Their shoestrings were made from ground hog hides.

Breaking cattle to the yoke, and ball games were Sunday afternoon diversions.

Whatever job at hand kept the boys busy: butchering, sorghum making, farm chores. No one could be allergic to work.

The younger children learned from observing their older siblings.

Hobart, Ottis and Mack were as full of notions as the branch was full of pebbles. They came up with the idea to fence in a "polecat ranch" near the spring. They staked it off and planned to dig trenches under the fence and put in 2 X 12 boards, so the skunks couldn't dig out. Alas! The plan died a-borning.

The brothers teased and "rassled." They hummed or sang songs as they played.

"Old Dan Tucker" was a favorite song. They played the Edison graphophone endlessly. They liked "Uncle Josh and the Dentist" and "The Preacher and the Bear." They knew all stanzas of "The Preacher and the Bear." Ottis would start the song; Hobart would sing the second line; Mack the third. They all joined on each chorus.

Excerpt From Childhood

On Sunday nights, the forbidden night for hunting, supper over and dishes washed, the Roberts family gathers around a roaring fire in the "big house." The children play games: Dominoes, Checkers, Fox and Geese, Hull Gull (using nuts); or they make a Jacob's Ladder design on their hands by using string.

They crack nuts they have gathered for themselves. "We'd go before breakfast to gather our caps full of chestnuts before the turkeys got them," Mack says. Someone brings in a bucket of apples from the "apple hole." "We'd eat a bucketful in the course of an evening," Mack says.

The children pop their own popcorn in an open-weave wire popper over the live coals in the fireplace after someone has shelled the corn by grinding two ears together between his palms.

Popperful after popperful of the crunchy, fluffy grain, popping like cap pistols, is emptied into a dishpan. The smell is tantalizing; they put away all of it.

Visitors are welcomed; they are news bearers. They carry neighborhood gossip from house to house. Mack tells of one old Union Civil War veteran, a frequenter. "He was an excellent yarn-spinner, but he didn't smell very good."

The boys never tire of hearing about Uncle Dickie's exploits.

"Tell us about that time when you ran into John Hunt Morgan." (Morgan was a Confederate general who led a cavalry squadron and executed a number of raids on Union lines in Kentucky and Tennessee.)

Uncle Dickie looks pleased. He takes a plug of Apple Tobacco out of his pocket, bites off a chew and works up a spit. He settles himself in his straight-back chair, and cracks his knuckles.

The boys sit on the floor surrounding him. Dickie begins confidently.

"Well, you see, we'd heard tell of Morgan and his goings on in our parts and they (Union officers) decided to do some scoutin'.

"Sgt. Ford, he offered to lead us. He picked 20 of us volunteers." Uncle Dickie takes a deep breath and puffs up like a toad.

"We saddled up our hosses and struck out. We rode quiet-like up the south side of the mountain. . ." Dickie moves to the edge of the chair, leans forward and looks at Papa and says, "We'd no more than got to the top of the hill 'til we run smack dab into Morgan's Raiders." When he says "smack dab" he pops his right fist into his left palm. Dickie sits back in his chair and crosses his legs. "Our leader, he says, says he, 'Spread out ... 'bout fifteen or twenty feet apart.'"—Dickie gestures, "'Wave yer guns and hats, holler loud and go after 'em,' but, says he, 'give 'em plenty of time to get away.'" Everyone laughs.

The raconteur uncrosses his legs, squares his chair, spits and begins again.

"We commenced to holler and charge. We created an awful racket, I reckon. We tuck 'em by surprise.

"Old Morgan he didn't know how many they wuz of us, you know, so he wheeled his hoss and hightailed it over the hill, and his bunch they all follered him."

Mack scoots closer to the narrator.

"We rid after 'em," Dickie says. "We wuz creating an awful

fuss, but we didn't foller 'em too far." Our reporter bursts into laughter. The boys join in; the father smiles. "They didn't fire nary shot at us, they didn't," he says.

"I can might near see 'em now," Uncle Dickie says and sighs. He rubs his right hand over his head and appears to be a hundred miles away from his admiring listeners, the smell of woodsmoke, apples and popcorn and the warmth of the fireplace.

"Did they run fast?" someone asks.

"Like a rabbit foller by a pack o' hounds." Everybody laughs again.

Uncle Dickie spits toward the hearth and looks smug.

"Were you scared?" another asks.

"By Drot, we didn't have no time to get scairt, buddy. No Siree.—'Course I doubt Morgan knowed they wuz just a handful of us.—And to tell the truth, we didn't know 'twas Morgan neither. Guess it's a good thing we didn't know." He grins broadly. "By Drot, you ought to seed them going over the hill."

He drums his fingers on a nearby table and appears to be in deep reflection.

"You know warn't 'till we got to—oh, I fergit the name of the place, that folks axed where wuz the rest of our bunch. We told 'em we wuz it. They liked to not a-believed us.

"Said they, 'you just run John Hunt Morgan's army off.'"

Dickie laughs again, rears his chair back, places his thumbs behind his galluses and looks pleased with himself.

Dickie shakes his head and seems to speak to himself. "Morgan could a gone through us like a dose of salts through a widder woman, warn't no use a runnin' off."

Uncle Dickie liked to tell about the time when his company bivouacked near Cumberland Gap.

"We didn't have no tents—nothing 'cept blankets. That night we all rolled up in our blankets and went to sleep. Hit snowed during the night. I woke up early the next morning, scratched out and looked all around—by Drot, my buddies all looked like a bunch of snow-covered logs."

Dickie was a strong Republican—strong as horseradish. He was terribly incensed by an editorial in our local weekly paper. He demanded that for the remaining duration of his subscription his paper be sent blank. The editor complied with his request.

During weekday evenings, the mother knitted wool socks or mittens for the family or sewed on clothes and quilts. She worked by firelight and lamplight.

Sometimes the fire made a sputtering sound. The Robertses called it "popping snow."

Home Life

The brothers used their senses like antennas. Motivated by curiosity, eyes filled with wonderment, ears attuned to the world around them, wants self-fulfilled, they imbibed the "tonic of wilderness." They grew in stature and wisdom.

The kids hunker for an hour at a time, fascinated as they watch two tumblebugs roll a ball of dung—pushing it along. The female lays her eggs in it, digs a hole and buries it. Why?

Another perplexing problem for them: why does a hog root forward for its food and a chicken scratch backward? And why does a hen cackle after she lays an egg?

They made false assumptions, too, as when Mack theorized, "Can't you fatten a mouse and make a rat?"

They were certain of one thing. The geese that paraded about as if they owned the farm were as effective as watchdogs in announcing a newcomer, and those webfooted fowls could attack from the rear.

The brothers learned the woods like a fox and passed through them as naturally. They knew which animal had made the track in the soil or snow—fox, coon, rabbit, or skunk.

They recognized the different kinds of trees as well as the different birds. They identified many birds by their song. If they didn't know the proper name of a bird, they made up one. 'Stacks' were little old sparrow-like birds that flew around the branch. The noise they made sounded like "stack."

Like their neighbors, the budding ornithologists collected bird cards. Every box of Arm & Hammer Baking Soda, purchased for a nickel, contained a small card with a picture of a bird in color. The card described the bird's habits, nests and song.

Communications

In the early part of the twentieth century children living in the country had access to few books. They had no movies, no radios, no televisions, and **no electricity.**

The Roberts family received the *Louisville Herald* at one period and the *St. Louis Democrat* for a time. Periodicals were limited to *The Comfort Magazine* and *The Progressive Farmer.*

The Gainesboro Telephone Company of Tennessee pioneered the telephone business in Wayne County. They maintained a central office in Monticello with party lines emanating into different communities. One party line might have ten to fifteen phones with designated signals for calling. Two shorts and two long rings, rung manually by winding the wall mounted telephone, sounded the Robertses' alert. (Mack also remembers that Mr. I. P. Shoemaker's signal was three shorts; Mr. O. C. Bell's five short rings.)

To call a friend on a different party line, one called through the Central office in Monticello.

One long ring connected the caller to "Central." "Hello, Central. Give me John Doe." Then everyone on both lines eavesdropped. One didn't tell secrets on a party line.

Before the invention of radio and television, storytelling was a great art.

The Roberts and Vickery families were taletellers. They laughed easily.

These stories gave the children a greater appreciation of their heritage. They helped shape their beliefs on morals, work, play and responsibility. What a happy household gathered around a flickering fire, parents sharing experiences with their brood and the children rapt in attention and full of questions.

A Baby Brother

Mack recounts: "One afternoon when we passed our Uncle George Orr's house on the way home from school, he came out and said, 'Boys you can spend the night with us; Rhodes said you could.' The next day we returned home to find a new baby." This one was a boy—Lisle. Now they were six—six sons! No longer the baby, Kermit tagged along after the older boys when he could keep up with them. Later, Harry, Kermit and Lisle were buddies.

The boys became self-sufficient fast; they had to. Of course, there were pets: crow, lambs, pigs. The pet crow "Loge" (Logan) learned to talk. When one said, "Hello Loge," he imitated them and laughed.

Loge showed fondness for bright, shiny objects. "He would fly down and get our pretty marbles when we played," Mack said. "Our mother had a little pearl-handled knife that she used for cutting button holes. Loge filched it. We found missing articles in Loge's treasure chest on the roof."

One afternoon the boys took a wagon to gather apples from apple trees scattered about the farm. Loge accompanied them. He carried his apple home in his beak.

Loge disappeared one Christmas Day. Hunters were in the neighborhood, and it was presumed they shot the crow without realizing he was a pet.

The Robertses raised sheep. Mack recalls his pet lamb, "Sheepie." "Even after Sheepie was grown," he said, "I could call him, and he would 'Baaaaa' and come." He didn't heed any other call.

"The lambing season was when the coldest nights came," Mack says. "It was a common sight to see my father light a lantern and go to the barn to check the ewes."

Sometimes a ewe died and left an orphan or perhaps disowned her own lamb. The lamb was then brought to the house and raised on a bottle.

Mack says, "My father told of a time when the University of Kentucky sent a man to Wayne County to demonstrate how much faster sheep could be sheared with electric shearers than the conventional hand clippers.

"'Uncle Tom' Kendrick, a skilled shearer, did most of the shearing in our county. He charged ten cents per sheep.

"The set time arrived. Farmers gathered at the Fairground to witness the match. Each participant placed his sheep on a platform. The 'Go'! signal was given. Using the hand clippers, Uncle Tom had his fleece off almost before the University man had started."

What a spectacle, Uncle Tom holding his sheep, now in its pink underwear, waiting for his contestant to finish!

Uncle Tom said he never felt so sorry for a man in his life as for the University representative.

Milestones

The second decade of the century proved to be memorable.

Woodrow Wilson was elected our 28th president in 1912. In that same year New Mexico and Arizona became our 47th and 48th states. The great "unsinkable" *Titanic* hit an iceberg on its maiden voyage and 1500 lives were lost. Mack remembers the tragedy.

The automobile became more visible. The self-starter replaced the hand crank that had resulted in so many broken arms.

Couples danced the foxtrot, and Puerto Rico became a U.S. Territory.

In 1913 an Amendment authorized income taxes. In 1919 the U.S. Congress ratified the 18th Amendment (Prohibition). The Woman's Christian Temperance Union, and others, greeted the news with joy. In 1933 the 21st Amendment repealed the 18th Amendment.

The Naming of (father) Rhodes Rankin Roberts

Mack Roberts speaks:

"Grandfather (Uncle Jackson) had a blacksmith shop. One day a drummer traveling by carriage came by on his way to McCreary County. He had had a breakdown and asked Jackson to repair the vehicle.

"Grandfather had had a son born the night before.

"During the conversation, as the buggy was being repaired, a bystander made a disrespectful remark about the stranger.

"The newcomer picked up a singletree from the shop and 'knocked the daylights' out of the rude fellow.

"Uncle Jackson admired the unknown person for his action.

"What is your name?" Jackson asked.

"Rhodes Rankin."

"I'm going to name my baby after you," Jackson said.

Grandfather Jackson Turns Republican

Mack Roberts speaks:

When my great-grandfather, Henry Roberts, moved from Virginia to the backwoods of Wayne County, Kentucky, he arrived a southern Democrat.

He had a large family, all Democrats, including my grandfather, Andrew Jackson Roberts, who was, no doubt, named for the president of the U.S.

My grandfather remained a loyal Democrat until the following occurrence.

Andrew Jackson Roberts had married and had several children. He was barely able to eke out a living on a small mountain farm. This was during the Civil War.

Grandfather Jackson had only one horse. One day, when he plowed with his horse, the Rebels came along and demanded the horse.

This was contrary to my grandfather's ideas. He protested. The Rebels did not argue. They beat grandfather brutally and took the animal.

When Jackson got his wits together, he decided the only way he could retaliate was to turn Republican. This he did. His brothers and sisters remained Democrats—but they hadn't been beaten and robbed of their only work animal.

The Country Store

Hobart, Mack and Ottis looked forward to the weekly three mile round trip to the country store. They went on foot and usually carried their coal oil can, spout covered with a small potato to prevent spillage. The kerosene was used in oil lamps and lanterns.

Just as the kitchen was the hub of the home, the country store became the center of the community. Neighbors came together to visit as well as to trade. They sat on nail kegs around a pot-bellied stove in the wintertime. They smoked, chewed tobacco, whittled and hashed over community affairs. Sometimes they played checkers.

Most everything could be found at the store: from mule harness to hotdrops; from cheese and crackers to chicken coops; from spring hats for ladies to shoe buttoners.

The housewife usually **sent** her eggs in a basket, to be bartered for needed supplies. In the summertime eggs could be worth as little as ten cents a dozen, in cold weather, as much as fifty cents per dozen.

Calico sold for five cents a yard; gingham sold for ten cents a yard.

At this market farmers bought their bibbed overalls, red bandannas, work shoes, hats and horseshoes.

Other obtainable items were kegs of nails, plows, axes and ax handles, hammers, saws, knives, boots, sacks of salt and wooden pails of candy.

Among the most needed items were thread 'ONT' brand was displayed in a glass-covered chest; each 500-yard spool sold for 5 cents), salt, crackers that were stored in open barrels, coffee beans shoveled out of a burlap bag with a shiny scoop, and .22 shells. Tobacco headed the want list of many households. No one in the Roberts family used tobacco in any form.

A can of salmon or corn might be afforded at the store plus some dried beans, if the home supply had been exhausted.

Farmers grew their own wheat for flour, and corn for cornmeal and hominy.

The store smelled of coal oil, leather, coffee, tobacco, cured meat and wood smoke—in wintertime.

A trip to the store served a double purpose. "Our local merchant was also our postmaster," Mack says. "We picked up our mail on our trips to the store." A stamp cost two cents, a postal card cost one cent.

The mail had been delivered by a carrier who rode a horse and carried the mail in locked waterproof bags. Not rain, sleet nor snow deterred the mailman. If a swollen stream proved unfordable, the mail carrier was still required to go to the rising creek and then return home.

When Mack's nephew, Milton Roberts, opened the modern Pic Pac Supermarket in our town, he asked Mack to speak at the ribbon-cutting ceremony. I remember among the other things he said: "A number of years ago, I made my first trans-Atlantic crossing by plane. I made the trip in six or seven hours. I wished I had had Christopher Columbus with me on the trip." It had taken him sixty-six days to make the same journey.

"Today, I wish I had my wife's grandfather, Uncle Lewis Bell, with me. I used to buy salmon at his store in Oil Valley—three cans for a quarter."

Mack continued, "I've cut over 4000 cords (umbilical) but this is the first ribbon I've cut."

The Aunts

In addition to his mother, Mack's unmarried aunts who still lived at home were his early female companions. They added a feminine warmth to his family life.

At that time, women dressed in floor-length skirts and blouses with choker collars. They wore whale-boned corsets nipped in at the waist. High buttoned shoes peeked from beneath their skirts.

"I remember," Mack says, "my aunts rubbed hops leaves on their faces for color. They wore "rats" in their hair. Rats were round puffs of store-bought hair that they placed over their ears. They covered the rats with their own hair pulled over the rats and attached at the nape of the neck. Bobbed hair was unheard of.

Back then a "fine woman" was a fleshy woman—buxom. The mania for slenderness was unknown.

The aunts entertained their beaus in a musty-smelling, lace-curtained parlor. A maroon carpeting added color. Couples sat on a horsehair sofa and visited or gathered around the pedal organ and sang—Aunt Lytha pedaling energetically. They usually sang religious songs such as *When the Roll Is Called Up Yonder.* They might end up with *Sweet Adeline.*

Aunt Ethel had tuberculosis. Aunt Lytha accompanied her to Colorado since the climate there was believed to benefit tubercular patients. They spent several months there. Aunt Ethel died a few months after returning home.

The aunts brought back a stereoscope with scenes from Colorado and the Rockies. Those pictures gave Mack his first glimpse of the outside world.

"My aunts brought me a little candy-filled pistol," Mack remembers.

"Aunt Lytha left home just before her father's second marriage. She lived with us until she married, except for a school term at Valparaiso, Indiana, where she obtained a teacher's certificate.

One summer Aunt Lytha worked at the old Seven Gables Hotel at Burnside, Kentucky. There she met her future husband, Charlie Snyder from Tennessee. He was a railroad tie inspector.

Grandfather Jackson had two buggies—black buggies, like those driven by the Amish.

The ladies drove a buggy to town, church or wherever. Sometimes they chose to ride horseback. They wore riding skirts and used sidesaddles.

One day Aunt Hannah drove the buggy to town; she left old Hawk hitched and the buggy standing! She had **eloped** with Carl André, one of the oil men from Pennsylvania. It is presumed they slipped off for the adventure of it. There had been no opposition to the match.

Someone had to go into town the next day and bring horse and buggy home.

The newlyweds went to Wolfe County where Carl worked in the oil fields for some time. They then returned to the Wayne County oil fields. Later, they migrated to California.

Mack missed his aunts greatly. They continue to live in his memory. Many years later, he visited Aunt Lytha, who had moved to Indiana, and his Aunt Hannah in California.

Mack Drives His Aunt Lytha to Town

Mack reports:

My Aunt Lytha, a spirited young woman, taught school 6 months a year. We lived in the same house with Grandpap Andrew Jackson Roberts. Aunt Lytha called me "Sonny."

My aunt taught me to milk. Today we milk Old Nell and Pied, two of the four milch cows gathered at the milk gap. This morning they wait to be milked and turned in to their calves on the other side of the fence. Another aunt will milk the other two cows.

Old Nell's calf has already been weaned, but the calves of the other three cows bawl and try to get through the fence to their mothers who chew on nubbins.

Aunt Lytha sits on a stool to milk Pied, but I stand to milk Nell. When learning to milk, I couldn't get a stream of milk larger than a pin, but with my aunt's encouragement, I got better.

Today Old Nell "holds" her milk.

"We might have to feed her some bran, Sonny."

"What fur?"

"Cats' fur to make kitten britches," Aunt Lytha teases.

We laugh. I like to hear my aunt laugh. Her laugh sounds like–well, like when the singing school teacher strikes his tuning fork on a table—'cept Aunt Lytha's laugh is a higher pitch and lasts longer. Or maybe it's more like when my grandmother rings her little silver bell. Everytime Aunt Lytha laughs, I do too, and everyone around her laughs.

"Bran" supposedly causes cows to "let their milk down." I feed Old Nell some bran.

"Ping, ping," then "swish, swish, swish," the warm, foamy milk fills my little tin cup; I empty it into a bucket and refill my cup.

"Saw," Aunt Lytha says when Pied steps her right foot forward. My aunt slaps Pied on the rump, causing her to return to a milking position.

Sometimes Old Nell swishes me with her tail. Puss, the cat, sits begging. I squirt milk directly into her mouth.

Smells of hay, corn, manure, cows and milk mingle with the fresh, cool air.

"Remember that new cow we bought, the one that didn't like women?" I ask.

My aunt nods.

"And when you hung your bonnet on the fence post, she butted the bonnet—Remember how funny it was?—and she kicked over your milk bucket, too?"

Aunt Lytha laughs. "You have a good memory for a ten-year-old."

My aunt fills her bucket and reaches for another. "Want to ride to town with me today?"

"You know I do. When do we leave?" I often accompany her on trips.

"As soon as we can get ready." Aunt Lytha begins to milk with both hands.

"Goody, goody."

While my aunt strips Old Nell, getting the last rich milk from her with a stroking movement of the thumb and forefinger, I leave to deliver my milk to the kitchen and get ready for our trip.

I put on my long-sleeved, blue chambray shirt, a pair of gray knee breeches Mama has made (I hate them) and the only pair of shoes I have. I wear the blue felt hat Grandpap Jackson bought for me when I helped him take the horses to town to be shod—the hat with the feather in the band.

I'm ready before my Aunt, who has to finish milking, strain the milk, and wash the milk vessels. She wears more clothing than I: a whale-boned corset, silk stockings, petticoats, waists and everything.

Aunt Lytha dresses like a lady. She is genteel—but not all prim like some women. She is lively; we have a lot of fun. I follow her like old Duke and Shep follow us boys.

I appear in the kitchen ready to go. My Aunt is about through with the milk things. "How would you like to do the driving today, Sonny?"

No answer is necessary. My smile tells all. "I'll get Old Hawk ready." He is one of the driving horses.

It is the trip I remember best because it was my first time to drive.

While Aunt Lytha dresses, I go to the barn, brush and curry Old Hawk to a fare-thee-well—until he's as slick as the ribbon on Aunt Lytha's red hat—the one with the dotted veil that she has laid out to wear. I harness him and hitch him to the buggy.

Old Hawk is a big, black horse with a white stripe down his nose. He is 16 hands tall—gentle and sturdy. He has made many trips to town.

I drive the buggy out of the barn and wait for Aunt Lytha in front of the house. My horse, impatient to get started, tosses his head, stomps, and nips on an apple tree. I'm eager, too. Aunt Lytha always buys me something when she goes to town—even if I'm not with her, she brings me something. I still have a cranberry and crystal mug she brought me from the County Fair. It has my name on it: "Mac 1905." That was the year of the Fair.

It's mid-October. The morning is brisk and breezy. Aunt Lytha comes out of the house humming, she is always humming or singing. She is all dressed up in a gray suit with a flounced white waist, her hat, and a pair of high-topped shoes. A gold watch is pinned on her lapel. She has painted her cheeks. She squints at the sky and says, "Fallin' weather." She often talks to herself. Aunt Lytha springs into the black buggy. She smells of lavender dusting powder.

I cluck to old Hawk and touch him with the long buggy whip that rests in the buggy whip socket on the front part of the carriage. He moves on down the lane—trots; that's his gait.

Aunt Lytha sits straight and proud on the seat beside me.

At the adjoining farm next to Grandpap's, the Mr. Perry Ingrams are shocking the ripe corn, tying it into tepees with binder twine. The field looks like an Indian village. The orange pumpkins that have grown along with the corn lie exposed in the field. Aunt Lytha raises a hand in greeting to the laborers. She knows all of them; I follow suit.

The road curls and we are soon at the Elk Spring, a spring that boils up from under a slope of a hill. "That's where Daniel Boone camped," my Aunt says. She's talkative today.

I know all about the spring. I've explored the area many times with my brothers.

At the Ingram residence half a dozen dogs run out and yap at Old Hawk's heels. He ignores them.

Past the residence and near the barn, a driver trains his trotters and pacers on a racetrack for the county fair. He is too engrossed in his work or play to notice us.

We rumble across the bridge that spans the creek from the spring. Sometimes when a tide is on, water covers the bridge and much of the valley we are approaching. Then we are isolated from stores, schools, churches and town—until the water goes away.

Farther down the road, a woman and her children dig sweet potatoes. The frail-appearing woman wears a bonnet. She wields a hoe as skillfully as a man. The children throw potatoes into a bushel bucket.

"That's hard work; poor Trannie," Aunt Lytha says and sighs. It's understood that women do the gardening. We wave to the workers. We see others engaged in the same task.

Old Hawk is really on the move now; mane and tail are flying in the wind. His shoes strike sparks on the rocks in the graveled pike. Dusty goldenrod and farewell-to-summer line the roadsides.

Sometimes Aunt Lytha clamps her hat with gloved hand to keep it from blowing off even though it is anchored with a hatpin.

I love to drive the buggy; the trouble is Old Hawk needs no direction—he knows the way already.

We clatter on until we arrive at the main road leading to town. Old Hawk stops and takes a left without my guidance.

A signpost says, "5 miles to Shearer Brothers Hardware." Old Hawk's "clip clops" seem to echo.

Aunt Lytha points out who lives where. "Now that's Uncle Lewis Bell's store and farm." She nods at the store on the left.

I'm familiar with the store. "That's where we take our eggs. That's where the peafowl are." I look for them. "We hear them all the time. They roost in the top of that big catalpa tree down there in the lane. Mama says when they call and carry on a lot it means it's going to rain. There's one now!" I point to a peacock as he flies upon the stile block. He thrusts his head up and down and lets out his strident call. "He's the prettiest bird in the world, isn't he, Aunt Lytha?"

"I 'spect he is," she says. "His feathers would trim a hat pretty, wouldn't they?" Aunt Lytha likes hats.

Across the fence a peahen pecks nonchalantly at the grass. "She's not as pretty as he is," I say.

"That peacock could have frightened Old Hawk," Aunt Lytha says, "but I reckon he's used to them. A while back, a woman from Burfield and her daughter were passing here in their buggy and a peacock strutted around right in the road-way in front of them. Just as the buggy got near—that bird gave out those awful shrieks and spooked the horse. He bolted and upset the carriage—wrecked it . . . ."

"The women?" I interrupt.

"Just scratched up a bit."

"Oh."

"Why do they have so many outbuildings at Uncle Lewis's? Is he kin to us?"

"No, Sonny, we just call him 'Uncle' because he is old and we respect him. Oh, the outbuildings—the log house back of the dwelling was used as slave quarters—before my day. Then there is the smokehouse, the chicken house, outhouse, apple house, buggy house, ice house . . ."

"Ice house?" I interrupt.

"Yes. It's like a cellar—below ground. When it's real cold in the winter, men cut blocks of ice out of the frozen ponds and store them in the ice house. They cover them with sawdust, then put a little house over them. The ice keeps milk and food cold until way down into the summer.

"Good idea. That's a good sweet apple tree down there in Uncle Lewis's Orchard," I point, "near that dug well. We stop there for apples on our way home from school."

Aunt Lytha doesn't say anything.

Now, mostly I just sit with legs dangling, taking in the sprawling valley that opens before us and enjoy the earthy smells and the jays jaying.

The woods that were so green a week or so ago have become colorful. Dry leaves skitter across the road. Cows and hogs wander freely along the roadway. Each farmer knows his own stock. There are no stock laws.

Hogs wear identifying marks: the Roberts mark is a swallow fork in the right ear (a notch in the point of the ear made by a sharp pocketknife) and an underbit (lesser gap) in the left ear.

A razor-backed sow roots for food in a roadside ditch. Small birds frolic and flutter taking their last meal before leaving for a warmer place. Horses stand head to tail in the shade. Chickens flutter across the road in front of us. A squeaky metal Lax Fos ad is nailed to a fence post. Our horse clatters on tirelessly.

Aunt Lytha and I discuss schools and teachers. "I wish you taught at my school, Aunt Lytha, I know you would be my favorite teacher."

"Now, Sonny, —"

I mention that the sky is spotty. My aunt calls it a "buttermilk sky." We laugh about that.

In the distance a flock of buzzards feed on carrion. More dogs run out on us. We bounce along to the rhythm of the hills and chuckholes in the road.

We meet a fancy double rig (two seats) drawn by a pair of fine horses. The two gentlemen riders raise their hats to my aunt. "Oil men," she explains, "probably going to the Denny lease."

"Where did they get those pretty horses?"

"From the livery stable, I reckon. They have them for rent, you know, and carriages, too—even drivers."

"I'd like to work at a livery stable . . . "

"And be a 'hostler'? That's what a person is called who takes care of horses at stables or an inn."

"I didn't know that. Yes, I'd like to care for horses and drive carriages."

Old Hawk keeps up his steady trot. We hear the sound of a motor and there, chugging over the bumpy hill right in front of us, is a machine running on wheels—an automobile; the second one I'd ever seen!

"Look! Look! Aunt Lytha."

"It's an automobile, Sonny. Haven't you ever seen one?"

"Once." I can hardly remain in the seat.

The automobile comes to an immediate stop. The driver, "Mr. Mooney—an oil man," according to my friend, shuts down the engine, gets out of the car, tips his hat to my aunt and leads our horse past the car.

Hawk doesn't appear to be very leery. He had met automobiles before. I turn in my seat and watch the car spin over the road until it disappears out of sight around a curve.

"There's not over a half dozen cars in the county, I reckon," my aunt continued, "but you just wait and see. Someday, I predict, they'll be as common as buggies—why you might even have one, Sonny."

"Who, me? Now, Aunt Lytha . . . ."

"You'll have one parked right in your garage."

"Garage" that was a new word to me. I didn't want to show my ignorance. When I got home my brothers helped me look up the word in a dictionary. "Garage"—a stable for an automobile. We also looked up "automobile"—a horseless carriage.

Aunt Lytha was always right about things, but this time, impossible. I'd never own a car, but I'd like to ride in one.

Hawk keeps up his regular gait—clipping along. He must be tired, but my aunt and I are having a good time.

We see women sitting on their porches.

"Resting before starting dinner," my aunt says.

Here's another signpost: "4 miles to Shearer Brothers Hardware."

More than once we meet empty wagons returning from delivering logs to Bassett's Sawmill. We also meet a woman carrying a basket of eggs to the store. With her are two pigtailed girls. They carry their jumping ropes and jump every few steps.

A washing snaps and flaps on a clothesline. It is mainly birdseye diapers. They dazzle in the sun.

We go over a little hill. "This is called Tuttle Hill," my aunt says. "That farm over there," she nods to the left, "is Mr. Will Elam's farm. He got it from Phil Tuttle.

"Right here, Sonny, that dilapidated log house on the right is where an important man used to live."

"Who?"

"A man by the name of Shelby Cullom. Now listen, he became governor of Illinois—served two terms and that's not all, he served four terms in the U.S. Senate—a man right here from our own valley.'"

"Never heard of him."

"See that big rock on top of Coal Bank Mountain over there? That's the Cullom Rock, named for that great man."

"Never heard of him. Who lives in that pretty brick house over there in the field? That house has seven chimneys. I've counted 'em many a time on the way to school."

"That's the Mr. T. J. Oatts plantation—a fine one, indeed."

"Why does he have so many mules in that field?"

"He fattens them up, and in the fall, his 'hands' drive them to Atlanta, Georgia. They auction them off to the southern farmers to use in the cotton fields. My, that would be a long distance to walk." My aunt seems to speak to herself.

Many unpainted houses with bare, unkempt yards line our

road—tenant farmers. Each laborer has his own garden and flock of chickens. More dogs rush out on us.

We pass a three-mile signpost.

"The next place is Mr. John Lee Ingram's," my aunt continues, "though you can't see his house from here. It's on the road that goes up by the Cullom Rock.

We travel on. Old Hawk is knocking off the miles—now we're at a two-mile signpost. "Whose farm is this?"

"Mr. John Oatts. The next farm is owned by Mr. Russ Oatts, the next by Mr. Charlie Oatts."

"Looks like, instead of calling this valley 'Oil Valley', they would call it 'Oatts Valley.'"

"It used to be called 'Coffey Valley' before the discovery of oil here. It was named for the Coffey family. Mr. Obie Coffey owned the farm now owned by Uncle Lewis Bell, and Obie's brother, Mr. Brandy Coffey, owned the land back of that farm and behind the Will Elam or Tuttle farm."

"Here's a one-mile sign. Shearer Brothers Hardware —"

"Now Mr. Leo Wright owns the big farm on the left," Aunt Lytha said.

In a short distance we arrive at the tollgate. Old Hawk stops before the pole barrier. The tollgate keeper, a woman, comes out of the house. She and my aunt chat briefly. Aunt Lytha gives her twenty cents. The woman lifts the pole that extends from the house across the road, and we pass through. The weighted pole is then lowered.

Now we are within the city limits of Monticello, Kentucky.

In the distance ahead of us, smoke rises from blacksmith shops.

We pass Bassett's Sawmill. I had gone there once with my father to deliver a load of logs. I remember that the mill foreman had shut down the mill so the workers could come out and watch Old Beck and Lou pull their load. We were proud of our team.

My aunt points to a white frame house on the left of the street. "Captain Tuttle's home—he served in the Union Army during the Civil War and was badly wounded, shot in the leg. The doctors meant to amputate his leg against his wishes. Capt. Tuttle told them if they took his leg off and if he lived, afterward he would hunt everyone of them down and kill them."

"Did they take his leg off?"

"No! They didn't dare. He walked with a considerable limp."

(Many years later, I heard Capt. Tuttle give the main address at the dedication of our Doughboy memorial.)

Before I have time to inquire more about the officer, I see Town Creek (Elk Creek) ahead of us. We pass around the bridge and splash into the rippling stream to let Old Hawk drink. He takes great slurps of the clear water. Of course, he is thirsty. Except for stopping at the intersection, for the automobile, and for the tollgate, he has trotted the entire seven miles.

Now we smell the acrid smoke we had noticed earlier. A rider sloshes into the stream. We drive away.

We are not the only comers to town this Saturday. Wagons, carriages, riders on horses are all around. "Almost like Court Day," my aunt says, referring to the crowd.

The sun has climbed higher. The day is getting warm. Aunt Lytha unbuttons her suit coat. "These dusty streets will be mud this winter, even miry. Over there, on the right side of the street, Sonny, the house with the gingerbread trim is Capt. Leander Jacob Stephenson's home, another Union soldier. I think he was wounded, too."

"Wonder if he knew John Hunt Morgan?"

"I'm sure he knew of him."

Now we were on my favorite subject, but we were also at the intersection of Michigan Avenue and a street that turns left (Church Street) to Mr. Charlie Hedrick's Blacksmith Shop and hitching lot. We turn. I pull my nag into the lot. It is jammed with buggies; we drive around—in and out, until a vehicle pulls out. I rein Hawk into the vacant space and loop his bridle over a post before you can say 'Christopher Columbus.'

Aunt Lytha opens her black leather satchel, takes out a looking glass and tucks a few wisps of her black hair under her hat. I stand ready to help her out of the carriage.

I hold her right hand. She lifts her long skirt with her left hand and moves gingerly onto the buggy step and dismounts. She brushes her suit with her hand, buttons her coat, straightens her hat and discovers one of the buttons on her left shoe is unbuttoned.

"I'll swannie, my shoe is unfastened."

"I'll button it for you." I know she would want me to; I've buttoned her shoes before. The problem was that 'gal squeezer' she wore. I'm raring to go. "Where do we go first?"

"To Miss Simpson's Milliners Shop, right up the street." As I said, Aunt Lytha likes hats.

We step onto a wooden walk, and I follow my aunt. Miss Simpson is a high-toned lady. She is glad to see Aunt Lytha. "I need a winter hat," Aunt Lytha explains to the hatmaker.

"But you wear fascinators (a light knitted woolen scarf women tie around their head) in the winter and a muff," I say.

My aunt pretends not to hear me. She tries on all sorts of hats. I like the one with the fancy spray of parrot feathers. My friend tries on every hat in the store 'cept a plain untrimmed hat. She buys a blue velvet hat piled high with black, flowing ostrich plumes—a pretty hat.

"To Shearer Brothers Hardware, next," my buddy says. "Pap told me to get some nails, and I'm afraid I'll forget them. Let's go now."

Shearer Brothers Hardware is on North Main Street. Aunt

Lytha propels me right along, though I turn my head like a screech owl, afraid I'll miss something. Aunt Lytha's heels click on the now brick sidewalk; her shoes creak.

My Aunt halts in front of the Monticello Banking Company. "Twenty thousand dollars total assets," she reads aloud. "My, my, that's a lot of money." She speaks to herself again, I think.

We cross the street to the hardware, and I come to a dead stop. "Look! Look, Aunt Lytha!" I gaze at the display of wagons and carriages. "That black buggy has yellow wheels!" I point at the vehicle. I'm beside myself.

My aunt leaves me mesmerized by the pretty buggies and goes inside the store to get the nails. Too soon she is back on the street. "Let's go." She drags me away from the store.

"I don't want a car, Aunt Lytha. They scare horses. I want a black buggy with yellow wheels, that's what I want." I walk backward, still admiring the carriage.

My aunt pulls me down the street. "To the clothing store next. Come on—Come on."

I reluctantly follow her into the clothing store. While she shops, I brace myself against the storefront window and watch the activity on Main Street.

What a bustle! Black laundresses carry balanced baskets of clothes on their heads. I knew they picked up the soiled clothes of the very wealthy, took them to their homes, washed, starched, and ironed them for a fee.

Carriages whisk by.

A wagon with a load of oil equipment, drawn by four mules, rattles down the street.

A grocery delivery boy jounces by in a one-horse wagon.

A team pulling a wagon catches my eye. Red tassels and red, white, and blue celluloid rings decorate the harness.

A rambunctious chap with his red cap turned backward

dangerously racks his slim, dappled horse among horses, pedestrians, wagons and all. He passes everyone.

A herd of brindle, roan, and pied cattle is driven toward the creek to water,—I suppose, by a driver whose straw hat has gone to seed.

A tall graying man with an Adam's apple carries his saddlebags on one arm. He is headed toward the Monticello Banking Company. He walks with a purpose. The hobnailed shoes he wears make a lot of noise.

A tottery old fellow walks with a limp behind a rickety, empty cart drawn by a bony mule. His check lines are around his shoulders. A burlap sack is across his arm. He yells at his mule constantly. A half-starved hound follows them. The mule gives out a loud bray.

A squat man, all dressed up in a suit with a gold watch chain across his vest, walks right by my window. He smokes a cigar. His celluloid collar looks uncomfortable to me. He wears a derby hat and carries a cane, though he doesn't appear to be crippled.

"Ready, Sonny?" Aunt Lytha interrupts. She takes a handkerchief from her pocket and erases the smears my hands have made on the plate glass window. "Fingerprints," she whispered. She nudges me out of the store.

"What did you buy?"

"A blue serge dress, face powder, hair pins, and other odds and ends."

Diagonally across the street, in front of the long balconied Ramsey Hotel, right under the sign that says, "Rates $1 a day," a little heavyset fellow with a mustache hawks apples. I'd seen him there before.

"Nice red apples—two for a nickel a piece," he says. I look up at Aunt Lytha. She smiles. We buy two.

Someone rings a schoolbell. For a moment I'm confused;

then, I remember that Mr. Lair, who owns a restaurant on the Public Square, announces that dinner is ready by ringing a bell. Grandpap Jackson and I had eaten at that restaurant once. We had the blue-plate special for twenty-five cents each, served family style.

"It's dinnertime," I say.

"We aren't hungry yet," my aunt says. "We can't stay in town too long. I'm 'specting company."

Amid the noise and confusion around us, I'm amazed to hear geese quacking and carrying on. I look at my aunt. She looks puzzled, too. "I swannie," she says.

Coming up Main Street, a young girl, a lad, and a man, each with long poles in their hands, are trying to drive a gaggle of geese right through the middle of town.

"Where are they taking them?" I ask.

By now, Aunt Lytha no longer looks astonished.

"I've heard farmers sometimes drive their geese to Burnside and ship them by train to Cincinnati. They are valuable, you know . . ."

"For their feathers," I butt in.

"Goosey, goosey gander/ Whither do you wander?" Aunt Lytha talked to herself again.

We watch until they come within close range.

"What's that black stuff on their feet?" I ask.

"Tar. They drive the geese through tar, then through sand, to put soles on their feet—so their feet won't wear out walking so far."

One goose wears a tiny bell. It tinkles like a fairy bell.

We aren't the only spectators. Children, businessmen, and women all watch, spellbound. A dog runs among the geese and creates a great racket, scattering them. The gawkers, including Aunt Lytha and me, close in and help the drovers regain control.

In the alley near the courthouse, a medicine man peddles liniment and snake oil.

"I'm hungry," I blurt out. "I'm going to eat this apple."

"Wait until we start home, Sonny. We're about ready to go. I'm having company tonight." She opens her pin-on watch, peeps at it and snaps it shut.

"Is it the doctor?"

She smiles brightly and winks at me.

I've heard the family tease Aunt Lytha about Dr.G_____. Someone said he is a "widower"—whatever that means.

"Guess I should buy my driver some peanuts and Cracker Jacks before we start home."

She knows what I like. She buys them at D. L. Tate and Son's Grocery where they have big bins of candy and all sorts of goodies.

"Thank you; you're good to me."

Purchases made, we return to the hitching lot, let loose our horse and climb into our vehicle. We retrace our way homeward, watering our horse when we come to the creek. We stop at the tollgate—no charge for return trip. I give our horse the free rein and eat Cracker Jacks and peanuts. I share with Aunt Lytha.

High clouds scuttle across the sky in front of us.

"My stars, these shoes are killing me!" my aunt says.

"Kick 'em off, Aunt Lytha—no one in this buggy but us; kick 'em off." I remember all the buttons—must be ten on each shoe. "I'll unbutton them for you."

"Please do."

At her feet in a second, I unbutton her shoes as I rock back and forth on the buggy floor.

Aunt Lytha removes her shoes. "Whew!" She lets out a big breath. "That's better. Now, if I had another thing off, I'd feel better. Reckon I can't do that."

I know she refers to her corset again.

I inspect the black patent leather shoes. "Where did you get these?"

"I ordered them from Sears, Roebuck; paid $2.10 for them; they were the fanciest shoes in the catalog, Sonny, 'worn by the latest prima donnas,' the catalog said. They have French heels," she brags.

"What's a prima?—Oh, forget about it."

My aunt smiles.

I find a whistle prize in my Cracker Jacks. I blow it and Old Hawk nearly jumps out of the traces.

"Maybe we'd better blow on the whistle after we get home," my aunt says, gently, and pats my knee.

The same dogs rush out on us, as before.

Now that we have eaten our peanuts and Cracker Jacks, I rub my apple on my breeches until it is shiny as a Christmas tree ornament. I bite into the apple. It is crisp, sweet, and juicy. "Try yours, Aunt Lytha. Best apple I ever ate."

"Hunger is the best sauce, Sonny." She polishes her apple with a lace-trimmed handkerchief. She takes a big bite, that is, for her; she usually takes little bites of food.

"You're right—delicious apple."

I look intently at my chum. "Why did that man selling apples say, 'Two for a nickel a piece?"

"Crazy, I guess. I'm pretty sure he's the man they fined for selling dressed rats for squirrels." Aunt Lytha frowns and looks disgusted.

"Eat rats! You don't mean it!" I'm all ears.

Aunt Lytha nods.

Now I **inspect** my apple. "It's all right, Sonny. Go ahead and eat it."

I don't need further urging.

We have been so busy eating and talking, we have passed the one-mile, two-mile, three-mile, and four-mile road signs without notice.

We approach the "five miles to Shearer Brothers Hardware" sign, where we will make a right turn toward home. "Oh my, we need some sugar. Pull off here in front of Uncle Lewis's store," Aunt Lytha says. She surveys the sky. "I do believe it's going to rain—we must hurry . . . lawsey day."

Again, I look for the peacocks. I don't see any. But guineas potracked and companied with the chickens in Uncle Lewis's yard. One Rhode Island Red rooster crows boastfully.

Uncle Lewis (who later became my grandfather-in-law) stands on the porch of the long white store. He gesticulates to a customer who is leaving. I stop the buggy. "Alight and come in," he calls cheerily.

Aged, bespectacled, small and wiry, he is ramrod straight. He wears graying chin whiskers. Uncle Lewis is a proper man— a gentleman. I never saw him when he didn't wear shirt and tie. He is ever ready to give the proper pronunciation of words, "according to Webster." A former teacher and Union soldier, he is now a merchant and a large landowner. Regardless of the weather, he can find a job for his hands. "Goodness, goodness, dock-digging needs to be going on," he laments.

"Did I feel a spit of rain?" my aunt asks as we dismount.

I hitch Old Hawk and follow my aunt into the store.

While Aunt Lytha makes her purchases, my eyes wander and read the signs on the products for sale: Wine of Cardui (for women), Dr. Legear's Laying Mash (for chickens), Grove's Quinine (for colds and malaria), Ring Ting Liniment (for rheumatism and sprains), Diamond Dye, Black Draught (laxative), Lax-Fos (laxative).

A Merry War Lye for hogs ad has a picture of a fine speci-men of a hog. He says, "I'm a Merry War Lye Hog." A little, puny hog beside him says, "I wish I was."

Aunt Lytha buys sugar—scooped from a heavy white bag, and carpet tacks "just in case" and we set out again for home.

A wind begins to stir; the sky darkens rapidly.

"Let him go," Aunt Lytha says, referring to the horse.

Old Hawk seems to understand. I loose the reins. Big drops of water begin to pelt the carriage and horse.

"My Stars!" Aunt Lytha says.

Our horse streaks over the graveled road toward home. He far excels his usual eight miles per hour. "I think he's going fast because he's hungry, don't you?" I look at my aunt. She nods.

"Probably. I usually take some hay for him, but I knew we wouldn't be gone long today." She smiles sweetly and has a dreamy expression. She sits erect and silent.

I know what's on her mind. "I'll air the parlor for you." I like to please her. I wait expectantly for her to reply.

She has a far-off look. "Are you going to fry a chicken for the doctor?" I'm hungry, again. I'd heard my mother say Dr. G_____ liked Aunt Lytha's fried chicken. I like her yellow leghorn legs, too. My mother said the doctor was the one who had suggested that Aunt Lytha go to Valparaiso, Indiana, for her teacher's cer-tificate.

"I think it's too rainy to dress a fryer, Sonny, and sometimes he's—he's on a call. . . ." her voice trails off. Again, she appears to be somewhere else.

I study my aunt curiously for a long time. Why doesn't she talk or laugh? "Aunt Lytha?"

"Oh." She turns, smiles, and gives me a pat on the knee. She straightens up and begins to hum a song. Now, she's back with Old Hawk and me.

We pass a woman driving her cows home to milk—in the downpour. It was a common sight to see Lou each afternoon head down the dusty road to fetch her cows that grazed by the roadside. Sometimes the cows had wandered as far away as three miles.

Today, trying to beat the rain, probably, she had gone for them early. An elderly woman, Lou always wore a black bonnet, an ankle length black dress, and a faded calico half apron. She travels barefoot. The rain drenches the poor woman.

"Poor Lou," Aunt Lytha said, sadly. "I'm getting this hat off," Aunt Lytha says abruptly. She pulls the hat pin out and removes her hat. Impulsively she takes the celluloid pins out of her coiled hair. She tosses her head; her black hair cascades and streams behind her. We laugh.

I take my hat off, too.

Puddles of mist hang on the hills like smoke from a moonshine still.

Aunt Lytha bursts into that ringing laughter again. I laugh, too—though I don't know why she laughs.

"Have you ever heard of Ichabod Crane, Sonny, and the Headless Horseman?"

"No. Why?"

"Nothing. I just think that's who we look like," she says and laughs that merry, catching laugh again.

Old Hawk makes a left and speeds up our lane, his mane and tail flying. He splashes mud puddles and spatters mud on the buggy robe we have pulled out to cover our laps.

Ottis, my brother, waits for us in the dogtrot. He dashes across the road and opens the gate to the barn lot.

The rain stops as suddenly as it had started.

I pull the buggy over in front of the yard gate to let my aunt get out.

She hoists her skirt above her knees and **jumps** out of the buggy. She brushes peanut hulls off her suit and dances a little jig. She picks up hat, satchel and shoes and walks toward the house. The dogs frisk after her.

Ottis and I drive into the barn shed and stable our horse. While my brother unharnesses Old Hawk, I pitch sweet-smelling hay into his hayrack with a pitchfork. Hawk begins to munch immediately. He sure is wet—sweat or rain? Probably both. I give him a parting pat.

My brother and I carry the purchases to the house.

Old Shep and Duke spring to meet us.

My aunt sits in a chair in the dogtrot. She has shed her dirty stockings. She chats with other members of the family.

"Aunt Lytha, are you sure it's too wet to dress a fryer?" I ask. "I'll catch it for you." I give her my best smile.

"What fur?" she joshes.

"Cat fur, to make kittens' britches."

Aunt Lytha laughs cheerily.

"I need to get out of these clothes, first, Sonny."

I know what item in particular she means.

I run to get corn so I can entice the chickens.

"I'll do the milking for you," I call back.

Springtime

Frogs in the branch announce the coming of Spring. This could happen during a letup of the cold weather in the latter part of February or early March. The sound always prompted the remark, "They'll be looking through glass windows yet."

Robins, home from the south, soon join the frogs; they come with the February thaw.

The boys are excited with robin's return. They watch him, resplendent in red vest and gray coat as he hops and runs, cocks his head and listens for a worm. All of a sudden, his beak strikes the ground and out he stretches an earthworm.

If March comes in like wild horses, that signals a bad month—but the boys aren't weather conscious. They might still find enough snow on a shaded hillside for a snowball, a compact snowball with which to pelt each other, or a dripping icicle hanging from a limestone ledge, to suck on. And everywhere is the sound of gurgling streams and the good smell of leaf mold. The boys soak up the magic.

Days and nights are equal now.

"It's sugar making weather," someone says, when he sees sap oozing from holes woodpeckers have drilled into maple trees.

"Frosty nights and sunny days are good for sugaring," Grandfather Jackson always said.

Mack uses a small ax to cut a wedge out of the side of a

maple tree. He hollows out the lower lip of the notch. The sap will gather into the hole. Next, with a brace and bit, he bores a hole into the bottom of the cup and inserts a spile, a joint of cane eight to ten inches long. He places a bucket underneath the spile to collect the sap. From eight to ten trees he obtains five or six gallons of the juice. Mack drinks some of the sweet sap.

He carries the clear, sloshing juice to the house and boils it in a kettle over an open fire in the yard. The sap is reduced to the consistency of syrup—his own maple syrup to be used on pancakes or hot biscuits with butter. Many times the mother used the sap to make cakes of maple sugar.

Buds begin to swell; cattle are allowed to range. The real signal of warm weather occurs when the boys hear the "honk" overhead of a harrow of wild geese homing northward. That heralded the time for the boys to shimmy out of their long johns, kick off their shoes and go barefooted. They loved to swish mud between their toes.

The grass grew green and the birds who had stayed around the fields and barn all winter eating seeds, were joined by those returning from the south. The trees wear a delicate green and squirrels twitch and frisk among them.

The world is awake; so are the Roberts boys. They sing:

> *Oh, a raccoon's tail is ringed all 'round*
> *An' a possum's tail is bare,*
> *An' a rabbit's got no tail at all,*
> *But a little bunch of hair.*

A New Sister

"One March evening," Mack says, "I realized that something was brewing at our house. Dr. Cook had been sent for.

"Hobart and a neighboring lady had ridden horses to church. Ottis and I were dispatched to get my Aunt Julia Orr. We accompanied her to our house. At her suggestion we returned to her house to spend the night. On our way, Ottis said, 'I think there's going to be a new baby!'

"Right he was! The next morning we returned home to find a new **sister**."

What a surprise and how happy the parents must have been. Just as the brothers who had arrived earlier had been welcomed, Joyce was welcomed and loved by all. She never showed any signs of being spoiled.

By the grace of God, the parents now had a brood of seven healthy children—Joyce being the youngest.

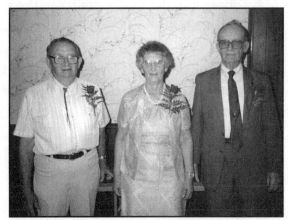

Lisle V. Roberts - brother, Joyce Roberts Logan - sister, and Mack Roberts

Farm Life

"Every farmer had a 'shop'," Mack says, "where he made or repaired many needed tools. He might make a 'singletree'—a wooden bar with hooks that fastened to the traces of a horse's harness—or shape ax handles and such."

Mack recalls, "We knew when someone used the shop from the noises we heard. We might hear the clang of a hammer sharpening a double-shovel-plow points that had been heated red hot."

As a child, Mack liked to turn the grindstone for his father to sharpen briar blades. He was fascinated by the shower of sparks produced, like a thousand fireflies, and the whirring sound where the metal came into contact with the grindstone. "But the high-pitched noise hurt our ears," he said.

By observing their father work in the shop, the boys learned repair work first hand. They were also useful. "Hand me a wrench," "Get the chisel," "Hold the other end of this singletree," or "Take a-holt of this 2x4," were constant orders.

Whatever the designated field work, the Roberts boys kept an eye on their father. They waited for him to pull out his pocket watch from his bib overalls, flip the cover of the Elgin watch open and announce, "Fellows, it's dinnertime."

That joyful declaration put a spring in the step of the worst laggard. Even the mules pricked up their ears.

Their traces are unfastened and the three small boys are hoisted, one by one, onto the sweaty, broad back of lop-eared

Beck or Lou, Kit or Lize, for the trip to the barn.

The harness jingles as the weary animals walk heavily toward their feeding place.

The boys are expected to hold onto the brass knobs of the harness. If they don't, and a mule stumbles, they tumble off— but they are tough.

After sipping gallons of water at the watering trough, the mules are put into individual stalls and left chomping on 8 or 10 ears of corn placed into each trough.

"Dinner" was the noon meal in the country. As the time draws near for dinner preparation, the mother, who has been working in the garden, picks up the baby from the pallet, puts him on her hip and goes to the house.

After placing the child in safe keeping, she stirs up the live coals in the cookstove left from breakfast preparation. She adds wood and tries to get the meal on time for her hungry brood and helpers.

In the early years of marriage, the mother had neither clock nor watch. In order to know when to serve the noon meal, she had made marks of the sun's shadow on the window sill, synchronizing the markings with the husband's watch. The marks had to be altered as the season changed.

Mack said, "My mother purchased her first clock—a mantel clock, after we had moved to the log house. She sold her turkeys and spent six dollars for the clock." It is still in use by the family.

Mother Roberts, with dinner well in progress and alert to timing the baking of bread, steps out of the kitchen and peers down the deep hollow. At a distance, she sees her diners coming. It appears that one mule carries a fly, another a bumblebee, and another a toad. Following them are the father and "work hands."

The laborers, eager to eat, march in from the fields wiping

sweat with red bandannas and fanning themselves with their straw hats. They wash at a handrail on the porch, where a bucket of water with dipper and wash pans are provided. Boys, as well as the work hands, wash with blue Lava store-bought soap. They dry on a white, coarse towel, usually smudged with little fingerprints, that hangs from a nail on a porch post. The men and boys comb and slick down their hair in front of a mirror on the porch wall.

Hungry grownups and children file into the kitchen and sit at a red-checked, oilcloth-covered table.

They relish the good, plain food: crispy fried side meat, green beans seasoned with pork and topped with new potatoes, corn on the cob, fresh tomatoes, cooked cabbage and onions.

A molded pound of fresh, yellow butter serves as spread for the hot cornbread or biscuits.

The "hands" pour their coffee from their cups into saucers to cool. They sip from their saucers. "Would you like cream in your coffee?" the hostess once asked. "No Ma'am, I take it barefooted," the man said.

Mack says, "Mama was kept busy refilling bowls, coffee cups and replenishing milk from a milk glass pitcher kept covered with a white cloth." The adults drank coffee; the children drank milk.

The diners glance from time to time at the stove where the opened oven door reveals a blackberry cobbler all bubbly and tempting. It will be served with fresh cream.

Lively conversation attends the disappearance of the delicious food. The diners eat with wooden handled flatware and three-tined forks.

After dinner, one of the boys takes his turn drying dishes. The other boys and men stretch out on the porch or under a shade tree for a nap. They cover their faces with their straw hats to protect them from the omnipresent flies. Rested, they return to the fields.

The mother breastfeeds or otherwise feeds her current baby. She diapers him and without any rest returns to her task.

"Our mother dashed from one demanding job to another," Mack says. "She ironed as she cooked since the wedge-shaped flatirons were heated on the stove top. Next, the churning had to be readied, the baby fed, and another big meal was coming up."

Young children's clothing was handmade. Mack recalls, "Mama made our breeches on her Elgin sewing machine, out of jeans—a cloth manufactured from our own wool. The breeches reached just below the knee and had elastic around the bottom." When the boys grew older, they wore overalls.

The older brothers wore hobnailed shoes—shoes with broad nails on the soles to prevent wear. Mack was never so fortunate to wear the unusual shoes.

A neighbor woman came in once or twice a week to help with the laundry. Rain collected in barrels was heated in a black kettle in the yard. Clothes were scrubbed on a wash board. Homemade lye soap was used during the earlier years.

Soiled clothing was boiled in the big kettle. Someone stood with a broomstick to punch down the ballooning clothes into the soapy boiling water.

Clothes were usually rinsed three times. Bluing—a blue liquid or powder—was sometimes added to a rinse water. It supposedly made clothes whiter.

On Mondays it was often a woman's aim to get her wash on the line before her neighbors. The Robertses, isolated as they were, didn't have to compete.

Tuesday was ironing day.

A farm wife needed enormous endurance. No wonder so

many farmers had two or three wives in succession—not because of divorce, that was almost unheard of, but because the wives died from hard labor. Such was the lot of women.

However burdensome the farm labor for the farmer, his heaviest load was usually the mortgage on the farm.

Farm Chores

Fuzzy faces, even so, by the time a son had reached the age of fourteen, he was treated as a grownup and given the responsibilities of an adult.

By now, big brother Hobart was entrusted to throw a "turn of corn" across the saddle of a nag, climb on and take it to the grist mill. There the corn was ground into meal—a staple, indeed. The brothers had helped shuck and shell the corn. They poured it into a long seamless meal sack. The miller took his "pay" out of a portion of the corn or the meal.

There was always a baby to mind.

One of the kids might be assigned as "water boy" to carry kegs of fresh water to the field hands.

The boys were constantly given orders, "Run and get the briar blade—and bring a file, too—and hurry," or charged to do any of the many tasks that were a part of farm life.

The Robertses, as well as their neighbors, used their own seed corn for planting. A mule-drawn corn planter dropped and covered the corn in a check-row pattern. Extra grains were planted to insure a good crop. Any unwanted plant was "thinned" (removed) by hand.

Corn-thinning time came when the sun was scorching hot and the thirst unquenchable. There were no shade trees in the cornfield. Mack says, "Sometimes when we pulled the top off the plant without getting the roots, the plant squeaked. We were then reprimanded by an elder to do our work right.

Children from the neighborhood were hired to help in corn thinning. One "cut up" boy would throw his cap as far ahead as he could. The kids raced in their work to see who could reach the cap first.

When the "corn thinners" paused to rest, they welcomed the sound of a red bird "whetting its strop." That sound was music to their ears; it signaled rain.

Always, among the children, there were the jokes and tricks played on one another. A sense of humor in that Roberts family came along with the name, probably as a result of the common genes.

Now and then they mixed fun with work. Mack remembers his Grandpap Jackson took him and his older brothers one fall day to the cornfield to chop corn stubble in preparation for wheat planting. Mack carried his own hoe. In due time a fire was kindled with stalks and Grandpap brought forth bread and bacon. They "briled" the bacon over the fire; nothing ever tasted better. Mack left the job after the cookout. He had lost his hoe in the meantime. "They always teased me about that."

Ears were ever attuned to the distress call of the robin, "gobble" of a turkey, "coo" of a dove, the cackling of a hen— bragging about laying an egg, the "cluck" of a broody hen to her biddies or her warning signal when she saw the shadow of a circling hawk.

Issues of social rights and non-rights and responsibilities stirred in the hearts of the little fellows when they saw a cowbird slip into a robin's nest and lay her egg. The irresponsible bird left the egg for the robin to hatch and care for. The robin pushed the offending egg out of the nest!

Churning

Churning was a despised task for the boys. "I hated to see Mama pull out the churn. I detested the time lost churning; that was a woman's job," Mack said, echoing the prevalent machismo, ". . . though I didn't mind eating a hunk of butter on Mama's crusty hot biscuits with jellies and sorghum."

The mother filled the churn about half full of rich milk. It had to sit until it "turned" or clabbered.

In the wintertime the churn sat on the hearth-side to hasten the process.

When the milk is ready, a dasher, a round stick similar to a short broomstick, with an X piece of wood attached to one end is placed in the churn. This dasher handle extends through the hole of the wood cover of the churn.

The dasher is pumped by hand up and down to agitate the milk perhaps for a half hour or so. At last, flecks of butter begin to appear on the surface. This butter is lifted from the buttermilk, worked in cold water, with a cedar paddle to give it form, drained and salted. It is then slapped into a wooden butter mold to shape it. The butter is then pushed out and placed in a covered receptacle and set in the cool water of the spring (in warm weather). The cold buttermilk is a favorite drink for adults.

There was an old saying, "You can't make butter when the elders are in bloom."

In fact, butter was often slow in forming. "For some reason," Mack says, "that prompted me to pour a little hot water in the churn. If that didn't work, you could put cold water in and churn another half hour."

The butter was placed in a glass dome-covered "butter bowl." The Robertses sometimes sold butter for twenty-five cents a pound.

Live and Learn

Mack dreaded to be awakened on a summer night by thunder. He knew the next sound would be from downstairs, "Boys, go to the spring [500 yards away] and move the milk and butter."

A heavy rain raised the water level in the spring and caused the milk and butter to float away, unless they were moved to a safe place.

A pair of drowsy boys pull on their breeches, light their lantern and start on their mission. The katydids are still didding. A clap of thunder shakes the earth and silences the katydids. A gust of wind extinguishes the light of the lantern. The boys grope their way up the hill and into the spring cove by flashes of lightning. They feel their way into the spring house and relocate the milk and butter.

Returning, big drops of rain turn into a torrent. The boys are drenched. Breathless, they get home and out of their clinging clothes and put on something dry. They snatch a gingersnap or two from the kitchen table and climb back up the ladder to bed.

The wind and rain beat in spasmodic gusts. The boys are soon fast asleep, unaware that the nearby branch roars and overflows.

Other than having to rescue the milk and butter, the sound of rain is melodious to our boys. "We knew if we got a good rain, the ground would be too wet to cultivate and we could go squirrel hunting."

During Mack's early years, when a neighbor became ill, someone went squirrel hunting to get a squirrel for the patient. For some reason squirrel was considered a delicacy—particularly the squirrel's head (brains).

This practice was perhaps Mack's first effort toward helping the sick.

Later, when they became strapping fellows, the boys had to forgo squirrel hunting on wet days. Instead they mended fences, shod mules or hauled timber to the sawmill.

"Before insecticides appeared on the market," Mack says, "on rainy days, flies covered the screen doors. Our mother reminded us constantly, 'Don't let the flies in.'"

In their Happy Valley, the brothers learned facts unknown to city children.

"Cut a notch in the base of your thumb nail to calculate the farrowing time of a sow.

"Three months and twenty days later, when the scar grows to the end of the thumb, the pigs are due to be born."

"To replace a broken ax handle, first remove the old handle. To accomplish this, we drove the ax bit deep into the ground— up to the handle at ground level. We burned out the old handle and inserted a new one." The bit had to be concealed, otherwise the metal would lose its temper.

"To cure a 'cracked toe,' tie a yarn string around it."

Observation: "Wild hogs cut grass and good-sized bushes and build beds before farrowing. 'Educated' hogs give birth anywhere."

Mack tells of his mother relating an incident that went back to the time when they lived with his grandparents.

The women were expected to keep a supply of spring water on hand. Grandpap Jackson liked "fresh, cold" spring water. Once he reprimanded his daughters for not having cold water on tap.

"If the house caught on fire," he said, "the first thing to burn would be the water bucket."

Toil and Pleasure

"For as long as I can remember," Mack says, "I could harness a mule!" He plowed when he could barely lift and shift the moldboard of the hillside turning plow at the end of the row. Hoofs and hands preceded tractors and combines.

In the beginning, this gave Mack a sense of growing up, doing what the older brothers could do.

He tells about using a plodding yoke of oxen, Buck and Dick, to pull a cultipacker in the White Gate field. Each field on the Roberts farm had a name. Other fields were called the Rye Knob, Ball Ground, Ten Acre Piece, the John Newground, Eph Thicket and the Carl Bottom. Mack walked on the left side of the yoke, holding a stick in his right hand. He used the stick to coax and direct the lumbering ox nearest him. The oxen weren't very good to use in hot weather—"They get too hot," he says. (Cattle don't sweat.)

Mack recalls plowing with Old Beck and Lou—a good work team. The Robertses had one mule named Kaiser—World War I vintage.

In plowing with a team of mules, the driver wears the checklines behind his shoulders rather than around the neck; his shoulders would be stronger than his neck if it became necessary to control the animals. The driver guided the team with one hand on the plowhandles and his other hand pulled the plow-lines in the direction he wanted the mules to go. He also controlled them by calling, "Gee," if he wanted them to go to the right or "Haw" to turn the mules to the left. "Get up" meant go. "Yea back" meant to back up.

"Our father required us to plow our growing corn four times—regardless. Sometimes the corn was taller than our mules; the white corn roots covered the plow points. Of course, this did more damage than good to the corn," Mack recognizes.

This type of farming utilized **horsepower**, in the literal sense, as well as **manpower**. Nothing was controlled by lever or button, but by patiently guiding the work animals and by following them **on foot**.

Mack continues, "We got our first three-mule **riding** plow in 1924. I liked to plow with it—it was such pretty work—each furrow the same." In using the new riding plow, Mack first learned that work was not work when he derived pleasure from it. That fact has sustained him for years and years in his profession as a healer.

When Mack was about fifteen years old, he helped his father and two other men drive a herd of cattle to Burnside. There the cattle would be loaded into a boxcar and taken by train to the Cincinnati Stockyards.

The twenty-seven-mile trip took 2 days. They took their Model T along. The first night they left their cattle at his Uncle Bolen's at Mill Springs and returned home by car. The second day they completed their journey.

When they arrived at the Big South Fork of the Cumberland River, they attempted to ferry the cattle across the river. They were unable to get all the cattle onto the ferry. The rest of the cattle plunged into the river.

"I thought sure we'd lost them," Mack says, "but the cattle swam across, following the ferry, with only their heads visible. We put them in the corral at the railroad yard. From there they went to market at Cincinnati."

The Newground

"Every year," Mack says, "just as surely as the year rolled around, there was a newground to clear."

After years of planting the same crop, usually corn, in the same place, the soil became depleted. This was before the era of crop rotation.

Farmers could not afford the little fertilizer available. To insure a good yield each year, they attempted to wrest from the forest a three or four-acre section, usually on a hillside, for a corn crop.

Throughout the winter on fair days the boys were mustered to help clear the land of trees and bushes.

The ring of the ax and the sound of the cross cut saws reverberate as a lofty tree is felled and trimmed of its branches. The majestic tree could have been there when Daniel Boone was a frontiersman.

If the newground is near the home, the logs might be used for a new outbuilding or cut into lengths for firewood. Otherwise, a log rolling is in order.

Neighbors are invited in to help with the project.

Usually four men handle a log, piling it into a heap with other logs and underbrush. A lighted match is touched to the tinder. The flame flickers for an instant, then ignites twigs and branches. Smoke billows, stinging the eyes. The fire crackles; flames leap and disappear. Sparks ascend a mile, it seems. Workers back away from the inferno. The logs are turned into ashes. Now the land is clear—free of its trees and bushes. With the pioneer spirit still in their blood, farmers thought nothing of denuding forests. Good logs were often burned. Timber was plentiful. Corn was scarce. "Conservation" had not yet become a household word.

Neighboring women come in to help prepare a meal for the occasion. They leave their babies lying side by side on a bed in the big house. They cook and visit. The meal is enjoyed by all.

Now that the land is deforested, a bull tongue plow is used to break the rocky, virgin soil. Stumps are circumvented.

When planting conditions are favorable, someone hitches a dependable mule to the bull tongue plow and lays off rows 3 $1/2$ feet apart. Then one of the women carrying a sack of seed corn follows the plow. She takes two steps then drops two grains of eight row yellow or white corn in the furrow at the tip of her front foot.

Another woman uses a gooseneck hoe to cover the grains of corn with two inches of soil. The men are busy overseeing the work, typical of the gender-based hierarchy.

During the growth season, the corn is plowed a few times with the same type plow. Weeds aren't a major problem the first year.

If good weather prevails, the first crop on the newground will be good. Because of erosion and the exhaustion of the thin soil, the productivity diminishes, thus the advisability of a newground yearly.

Corn was a vital crop, useful for livestock as well as man. Considering how much grain the mules and horses ate, the Roberts boys often wondered who worked for whom.

The tractor had not yet been invented. Anyway, the gas guzzler would have been useless on the hillsides.

Mack still has a vivid memory of seeing a neighbor tend a

poor newground. The man walked behind a bull tongue plow pulled by a jenny (a female donkey), "not bigger than a rabbit."

Now when Mack visits his homeplace, he can't believe how completely nature has reforested the newgrounds they had cleared so recently (it seems to him) though it has been seventy-five years. Once again, those plots are woodlands, filled with mature trees.

Fertilizer

Horse, cow and chicken manure, though insufficient, served as fertilizer for the small farmer in the early part of the twentieth century.

Mack said, "My father had heard of commercial fertilizer. He had been told that if one rubbed fertilizer on his shoe soles and walked across a pasture, he could be tracked by the greener growth in his footprints."

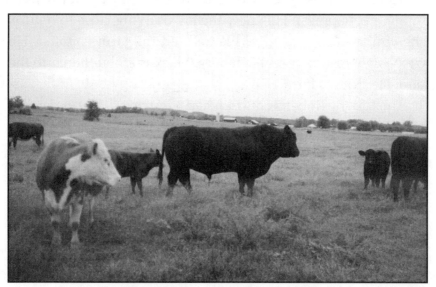

Dr. Roberts's bull at his Mill Springs farm.

Industry

Farming ran deep in the Roberts family blood. All six sons became farmers. Could that tendency have been the result of shared genes? True, many of them entered professions also, but one wonders if farming might have been their first love had it been more rewarding financially.

I hear of many of the same generation with similar backgrounds who fled that life style and wished to wipe it out of their memories. They became part of an exodus to the city seeking a "better life."

To Mack, those memorable early years on the farm were among his happiest. He knew the joy of living close to nature. The young farmer realized his help on the farm counted. He saw visible results from his labors. Mack is still tethered to the land. He owns a farm.

Though the Roberts children had a restricted, isolated childhood, they had a fulfilling one. They had God-fearing parents and entertaining siblings. Farm work hardened their muscles, and fostered ingenuity, cooperation and self-reliance. By the time they had left the sanctity of the home, their opinions on most things had crystallized from those impressionable years.

They lived by the "code of the mountain" when a man's word was his bond. A man who would not work or pay his debts was an outcast.

Homes had no locks on them.

Materialism had not yet triumphed.

God reigned in their hearts.

Life was unhurried.

Through their wholesome surroundings, removed from many temptations, they got a perspective that is lacking in the lives of present-day children who have been brought up in a permissive society.

It would be erroneous to characterize their early years as spent in poverty and poor circumstances. The Robertses were quite as well off as their neighbors—average middle class.

Their economic situation depended upon the bounty of the cultivated fields and forests, and that was contingent upon the weather and effort expended.

The Robertses were recognized in their advanced farming practices. They had the first silo in the county.

All seven of the children were high school graduates. Five were college graduates—unusual for a middle-class family in Kentucky during the first three decades of the 1900s.

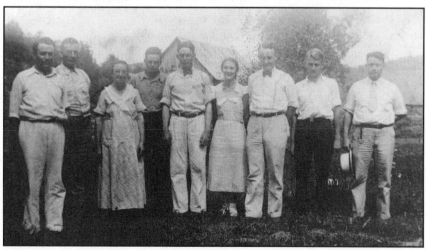

Roberts Family. (left to right) Hobart, parents—Rhodes and Rona, Kermit, Harry, Joyce, Mack, Lisle and Ottis.

School Days

Mack entered the Oil Valley School at the age of six. The one-room building was a distance of 3 1/2 miles from his home.

The barefoot children walked the dusty road until frost. The short winter days forced Hobart, Ottis and Mack to ride Old Lottie, a mare, part of their mother's dowry, to school (no school buses).

The bare school room had double desks. A blackboard lined the front wall. A well supplied water. They had **no electricity**.

One teacher taught all eight grades. Enrollment sometimes reached up to sixty pupils. The school year extended from July until Christmas; school hours stretched out from 8:00 a.m. until 4:00 p.m.

Pupils were allowed to attend grade school until they were twenty-one years old. Many repeated the eighth grade three or four times since this concluded the schooling for the majority of them.

The teacher arrived at the school with bell, broom, chalk, water bucket, dipper, coal bucket, shovel and record book—all dispensed by the county superintendent's office.

If fortunate, the teacher might find her assigned school has a library consisting of a dictionary and a half dozen books— among them *Robinson Crusoe*, *Pilgrim's Progress*, and perhaps *David Copperfield*.

On Mack's first day at school, he shared a desk with his older brother Hobart. When Hobart received permission to go to the well to get a drink, the little beginner, holding his new tin drinking cup, ran after him.

"Come back here, little man, and walk out," Mr. Obie Ryan, the teacher, ordered. That marked the end of the school term for Mack. He never returned to school.

The next year, Miss Amanda Lovelace was his teacher. As teacher's pet, he completed the school year.

Other grade school teachers were Mrs. Linnie Davis White, Mr. Willie Shearer, Mr. Adron Back, Miss Hettie Long, Miss Alta Saunders, Mrs. Bess Dalton Stokes, and Mrs. Jennie Stone Elam.

Mack voluntarily remained in the third grade for a couple of years. He doesn't remember why.

"Keeping order" was the main criterion for judging teachers. "Spare the rod and spoil the child" parents supported the teachers. Indeed, the one who taught them to get out of bed when called and the one who drilled them in the multiplication table were usually in alliance. If you got a whipping at school, you got one from your parents when they heard about it. Needless to say, an enviable learning atmosphere prevailed.

School Experience

Each teacher laid down the law at the beginning of the school term, prohibiting such antics as throwing paper wads. When the teacher turned his back, some scamp acted up only to find the teacher had eyes in the back of his head.

The offenders could be subjected to a humiliating punishment. For example, one might be required to stand on tiptoes at the blackboard with his nose in a chalk circle drawn by the teacher, for a specified length of time.

Most schoolhouses of the era had outhouses. The woods were

accessible at Oil Valley and served the same purpose.

To be "excused" the pupil held up his hand and asked permission from the teacher. With consent granted, he would leave a book lying on the floor by the door as evidence that one person was out of the room—a requirement.

Teachers, by virtue of their position, were custodians of the schoolhouse. Sometimes, some fortunate boy was given the daily job of starting fires or sweeping the schoolroom for the enviable sum of fifty cents a week.

One year Mack got a fifteen-cent Barlow knife for not missing a day at school.

"Rrring - Rrring!" the teacher summoned the children to "books" with a hand bell.

"How old are you, Johnny?"

"Six years old, going on seven," he answered.

The teacher called the pupils in the class being taught to the "recitation bench" in front of the room. Everyone in the room, if attentive, profited from whatever was presented in a higher grade—probably by osmosis.

Recesses were the most fun, particularly noon recess. When "recess" was announced, all kids tried to leave the room simultaneously, unless restrained by a strict teacher.

"We hastily ate our basket lunches of fried chicken, fresh tomatoes and all sorts of goodies," Mack says, "in order to play Fox and Hound, Town Ball, Marbles, Mumblety-peg, or whatever. Many times we pitched horseshoes or jumped red pepper on a grapevine jumping rope."

The kids had no physical education classes. After having walked the seven miles round trip to and from school, plus playing at recess, and afterward doing farm tasks when they arrived home, they had exercised enough.

They enjoyed the long walk with a road full of other children. They feasted upon tempting apples dangling from trees across the fence. There were persimmon, hickory nut, walnut and chestnut trees to be raided. In cold weather they skated on frozen ponds.

Often courting couples lingered behind. They preferred not to walk with the crowd.

Many of the boys developed real marksmanship by throwing at birds resting on a limb or at the green insulators on telephone poles! Mack says, "Garnett could 'bust' one fifty yards away—with his left arm.

"Sometimes when we were caught in a rain going home, our father would meet us with dry coats."

An embarrassing incident once occurred during the shorter days when the three boys rode a horse to school. The riders overtook some of their walking classmates, among them Hobart's girlfriend. Just as the boys passed their friends, the smitten boy switched Old Lottie to get her to trot. Lottie jumped and spilled all three kids, much to the embarrassment of the young suitor.

"I rode in the middle," Mack says. "They accused me of pulling them off."

"We always turned our horse loose at school," Mack says. "She wouldn't stay hitched. She stayed around until time to go home. We carried corn in the saddlebags for her lunch."

Studies were interrupted when the boys were kept home to cut and gather corn, put up hay, or to help with butchering or sorghum making.

"Frequently on Friday afternoons we had a spelling bee," Mack says. Anyone could participate. Pupils lined up and the teacher pronounced the word to be spelled.

"The pupil repeated the word, then attempted to spell it. If we spelled the word correctly, we kept our position in line. If we missed the word, the next person in line to properly spell the word 'turned us down' and moved ahead of us. The last person left standing won the contest."

Once in a while, the teacher asked an upperclassman to listen to a first or second grader read, or pay attention as a third-year kid chanted the multiplication table.

Mack remembers one time when he gave out spelling words to Walter. "Spell 'coo.'"

"C-o-double o," Walter said.

"Correct" his agreeable teacher announced. He knew the correct spelling; he also understood what Walter meant.

Friday afternoon was sometimes devoted to debates such as "Who was greater, President Washington or President Lincoln?"

Many Fridays following afternoon recess, the children were allowed to just sing. A favorite selection was, *Row, Row, Row Your Boat.* They sang the song in "rounds"—that is, the singers were divided into groups in which the second group starts singing when the first group reaches the second phrase—and so on.

Among other favorite songs were *America; Darling Nellie Gray; Long, Long Ago; When You and I Were Young, Maggie; Auld Lang Syne; Yankee Doodle; Massa's in the Cold, Cold Ground.*

"Miss Jennie," Teacher Extraordinaire

For four years Mack was privileged to have a well-known grade school teacher, Miss Jennie Stone Elam. She taught all eight grades in the one-room school.

Though hardly five feet tall, she was stocky and straight as the pencil she wore over her ear in her short, curly, auburn hair.

A noted disciplinarian, Miss Jennie's punishment came with the charge—instantaneously by a switch. (The culprit was sometimes sent to the woods to get the switch to be used.) She instilled fear even in the grownups.

The schoolroom is a working world. The only sounds are the soft whispers of a pigtailed girl mouthing words to herself as she runs her finger under a line in her primer, the whir of a wall-mounted mechanical pencil sharpener when a small boy grinds away his cedar penny pencil. He stares out the window at a sow rooting in the school yard. A fly buzzes in the unscreened window.

The pupils freeze in terror when their teacher patrols the aisle. They hold their books in front of them and appear studious. Their eyes follow the teacher. One snap of her finger and one could hear a ghost breathe.

Jim tells of his first day at school in Miss Jennie's classroom. She walloped him good, though he had not misbehaved. "That's for your brother, J. D.," the teacher told him. J. D. had been her pupil the year before. Evidently, J. D. had been a bit of a problem. The "school marm" instilled fear in Jim, who still curses every time he tells about the incident.

"She would flog you for looking impudent," a former student says.

Miss Jennie set Mack on his course and had a great influence on his life. She favored boys.

She not only taught the "scholars" the 3 R's, but the submissive children received instruction in the social graces. Mack says, "She had us tipping our caps to every lady we met. We were taught to remove our caps or hats when we entered a building. She taught us how to make introductions. She instructed us not to enter a church or classroom while someone read from the Bible."

Furthermore, their teacher taught the boys to open their pocket knives (most boys carried a Barlow knife) for a girl who asked to borrow the knife to sharpen her pencil. They extended the knife to the girl, handle first.

Under Miss Jennie's tutelage, Mack received an outstanding background in grammar and literature. "We learned to diagram sentences until we could do them in our sleep," he says. (He is my grammarian.)

Mack tells about the time when studying "gender," a boy was asked the gender of "cat."

"Show me the cat," the boy said.

"We had to memorize every poem we came to in our Readers," Mack adds. He has a great love and enviable knowledge of poetry.

Some fifty years later our daughter Ann had Miss Jennie for her fifth grade teacher in the Monticello Independent School. She, too, was in awe of her instructor but liked her.

"On the first day of school," Ann says, "our teacher assured us that 'Every pupil in the room will make an A on deportment. Otherwise, it would be a reflection on me.'" And so they did!

Ann gives an example of one of Miss Jennie's visual aids. "She took a tin can, the kind that sits on top of a stove to supply humidity to a room, and turned it upside down.

"'I inverted this can,' the teacher said, 'to divide fractions, you invert and multiply.'"

A rabid Democrat, Miss Jennie was vocal about politics as well as community affairs.

She could be fun, too. Most of her pupils finished the school year fond of their teacher.

Curriculum and School Experience

"We used the McGuffy Readers at Oil Valley School," Mack says. Those classic volumes were filled with works of literary geniuses such as Irving, Whittier, Lamb, Byron and Defoe. They were a great source of extraordinary adventure, clever fables, and beautiful poems. Mack has a set of the readers now and peruses them from time to time with apparent enjoyment, often reading the poems aloud.

Geography received great emphasis. "We were required to give the bounds of each of the 48 states (at that time), draw the map, learn the capital and leading industry of each state. Children also had a global awareness.

Spelling and physiology were both stressed. Penmanship was overlooked—as Mack's writing attests.

History, particularly American history, was significant according to the teacher. Interest begets interest.

Mack recalls a trip he made as Wayne County Health officer to a school in a remote part of the county. There he was to immunize children against smallpox, diphtheria and typhoid. "I had two more schools to visit that day, but my nurse and I had to sit down in the classroom and wait for Mr. Greene to finish teaching the American history lesson.

"That teacher marched General Burgoyne all the way from Canada by the way of Lake Champlain and Ft. Edward to Albany, New York. General Howe was expected to sail up the Hudson from New York, but before doing that, he planned to march across New Jersey to capture Philadelphia.

"Washington's Army stopped General Howe a couple times and caused him to be too late to help Burgoyne. Thus, Burgoyne had to surrender to General Gates at Saratoga."

We visited those sites a few years ago. This took Mack back to his school days with Miss Jennie. "She had us tracing armies all over the country," he said.

Indeed, his travel experiences have helped him crystallize what he had learned. His background had stirred his interest; travel brought it to life. The setting for history and the poems he memorized are part of him.

Mack easily mastered arithmetic, a Roberts characteristic. The grade school children pondered such problems as which is heavier and how much: a pound of feathers or a pound of gold? A pound of feathers weighs more than the pound of gold, derived from the fact that the weight of feathers is computed on the avoirdupois scale, sixteen ounces to the pound, whereas gold is computed on the Troy scale—twelve ounces.

Mack still remembers that a twenty-four inch by twelve foot log contains three hundred board feet.

Brain teasers intrigued the kids. "If a hen and a half can lay an egg and a half in a day and a half, how many eggs can six hens lay in seven days?

Another perplexing problem made the rounds regularly. A man needs to cross a stream. He has with him a fox, a goose and a bag of corn. He can carry only one item along at a time. If he leaves the fox with the goose, the fox will kill the goose and eat her. If he leaves the goose with the corn, she will eat the corn. How can he solve his dilemma?

There were always pranks in the classroom. A large coal or wood burning stove heated the room in cold weather. The kids had a habit of surreptitiously placing chestnuts on the stove to roast during "books." Often times a chestnut exploded causing a loud noise. No one ever claimed the chestnut. Chestnuts were plentiful before the devastating chestnut blight of the 1920's.

The children were not deterred from attending school by rain, sleet nor snow.

Mack says, "No one ever suffered from the stern discipline. We learned when we entered school that we were expected to 'learn'—and learn we did!"

Those were the formative years.

Winter Schools

After the conclusion of the regular school term a teacher might teach a "subscription" school for a few months. These winter schools were open to anyone who subscribed for a certain fee.

Moonlight Schools

Moonlight schools were government sponsored. They were taught at night by teachers who gave free service to teach the illiterate. Many elderly people took advantage of this opportunity.

Mack tells of a neighbor who attended the school and learned to write his baby's name. "He just beamed." The moonlight school had been his first chance to learn to read and write.

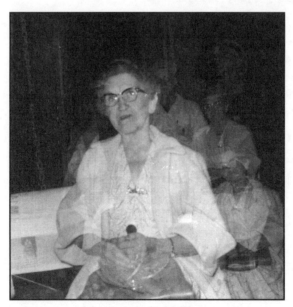

Mrs. Jennie Stone Elam.

Teacher's Examination

In the early decades, the twentieth century teachers qualified for their positions by passing a teacher's examination, sent out by the State Board of Education. First, second and third class certificates were issued, depending upon test scores. Many teachers prepared for the examination by taking courses at a local Doublehead Academy owned and operated by the Mr. Frank Shearer family.

Teacher's Examination

Courtesy of Betty Shearer Caylor

SPELLING:

Q. Use the following words in sentences: (a) supersede, (b) subterranean, (c) conjecture, (d) demeanor, (e) apprehend, (f) theorist, (g) cardiac, (h) beneficent, (i) equable, (j) clandestine.

Q. Mark diacritically the words supersede, etc., in above question.

READING:

Q. Give a brief but concise account of the Montessori Method.

Q. How may and should a teacher direct a class in the reading habit?

GRAMMAR:

Q. Analyze the following sentence and classify with respect
to meaning and forms:

> "There is a reaper whose name is death,
> and with sickle keen,
> He reaps the bearded grain at a breath,
> and the flowers grow between!"

Q. Discuss the value of conversational exercises in grammar.

COMPOSITION:

Q. Write a letter to one of your patrons relative to the absence
of a pupil and emphasize the importance of his attendance
at school.

Q. Write a composition on some subject to be chosen by the
County Board of Examination.

WRITING:

Q. Write a letter making application for a school as a speci-
men of your penmanship.

Q. Copy the following as a specimen of your writing:

> "Within the shade of elm and oak
> The church of Berkley Manor stood:
> There Sunday found the rural folk,
> And some esteemed of gentle blood.
> In vain their feet with loitering tread
> Passed 'mid the graves where rank is naught:
> All could not read the lesson taught;
> In the republic of the dead."

Alma Roberts

ARITHMETIC:

Q. A circular pond is 100 feet in diameter with ice 8 inches thick. Find the number of tons of ice on the pond, if a cubic yard of water weighs 1687.5 lbs., and the specific gravity of ice is .9.

Q. Add to 4.025, 13.12, subtract their difference and multiply the remainder by the quotient of difference divided by .004.

PHYSIOLOGY:

Q. What is the alimentary canal? Name its different parts.

Q. What are the functions of (a) fat, (b) saliva, (c) synovia, (d) sweat, (e) tears, and (f) muceous?

HISTORY:

Q. Explain the effect of the colonization of America by different foreign nations upon the character of our political and social institutions.

Q. What was the condition of this country at the close of the Civil War?

LITERATURE:

Q. Name four American historians and give work of each.

Q. Who wrote: (a) *A Blot on the Scutcheon*, (b) "The Mansion," (e) *In Memoriam*, (d) *Treasure Island*, (e) *Westward Ho*, (f) *A Child's Garden of Verses*?

Q. Give the authors of "Lycidas," "Le Morte D'Arthur, Essays of Elia," "Locksley Hall," *Marmion*, and *Our Mutual Friend*.

GEOGRAPHY:

Q. Discuss: "In the different stages of a child's life are reproduced the stages of civilization."

Q. How ma[y] geography, history and civics be correlated? Give your plans in brief.

Q. Give the qualifications of a voter in Kentucky.

Q. Distinguish between the Federal Government and the State Government.

THEORY AND PRACTICE:

Q. Is teaching a profession? Why?

Q. If the trustee should criticize you severely for what you know to be your duty, what would you do then and afterward?

School Programs

Christmas Programs

Christmas programs created great excitement for the school children as well as for the community.

A few days before the program, the teacher commissions some of the older boys to scout out a tree for the classroom. Regardless of accessible trees, usually cedars, the boys make it an all day project. They take turns chopping until the bushy tree falls with a thud.

They search out mistletoe, with berries looking like blisters. If they can't climb the tree where the mistletoe is found, they shoot the mistletoe out with a rifle. They also bring in prickly-leafed holly. Branches of these two evergreens are usually placed in windows or vases.

The tree is always too tall and has to be trimmed just so the tip of the treetop allows room for a star. The star is covered with tinfoil from tobacco wrappers.

The Christmas spirit arrives with the tree. The schoolroom smells like Christmas. Joy and gladness fill the hearts of all. Older and younger kids join in decorating the tree and classroom.

Chains are made from red and green construction paper and glued together with paste. They are used to encircle the tree along with tarnished tinsel.

Strips of red and green crepe paper, with edges stretched at intervals to give a ruffled effect, are crossed diagonally below the ceiling. A red accordion folding type bell is hung at the intersection.

Popcorn popped on the heating stove is strung by needle and thread to loop around the tree. The tantalizing popcorn is irresistible and much of it never graces the tree.

In the school yard, during recess, ears are assailed by the loud "bang" of nickel fire crackers or the rat-a-tat-tat of a string of penny firecrackers. The sputtering of a Roman candle exploding and discharging sparks and balls of fire creates more excitement.

Pupils "draw names" a week or so before the Christmas program and exchange gifts.

Gifts are tied on the tree. Handkerchiefs are popular items. Since many of the students are in their late teens, they sometimes put rings or wrist watches on the tree for sweethearts.

Every child participated in the Christmas program, having a "piece" to say or a "play part."

Mack still remembers the beginning of one verse repeated yearly by a boy who had long outgrown the poem:

> Along about this time of year
> Seems I get to feeling queer.

Among the songs sung were *Jolly Old St. Nicholas, It Came Upon the Midnight Clear,* and *Jingle Bells.*

Of course, Santa Claus made his appearance and gave out gifts.

Christmas and the end of the school year came at about the same time.

The Community Box Supper

A money raising event for the school was the box supper.
Young ladies in the community decorated boxes containing

the best supper-for-two their mothers could prepare. They did this to favorably impress the wished-for buyer. This tested the prowess in the kitchen of each participating housewife. The identity of the owner of the box is unrevealed.

The auctioneer, a colorful community man, offers the boxes to the highest bidder.

The familiar chant: "I'm bid thirty. Now, who'll make it forty? Forty. Who'll make it sixty? —Come on, fellows, the girl who prepared this box is beautiful and a good cook like her mother . . . ."

The successful bidder, a young swain who may have used devious means to ascertain whose box he bids on, not only gets to eat with the fair lady but also may be fortunate enough to walk her home.

Box Suppers often proved to be matchmakers.

A "Pretty Girl Contest" follows the selling of the adorned boxes.

Girls who have admirers are nominated for "The Prettiest Girl." This behooves the fellows to put their money where their hearts are. The winner usually receives a box of candy.

Money earned from these affairs was used to purchase school supplies.

Once in a while a "shooting" occurred at Box Suppers. Moonshine was readily available and many men carried guns.

Mack recalls an incident when a teacher was killed by a drunk's firing into the crowd.

At another Box Supper in a remote part of the county, two drinking buddies collaborated and bought every box offered. They paid for the boxes, accepted none of them and, in pursuit of more fun, left the school—and many disappointed girls.

School "Marches"

Probably to break the monotony of the non-social season or just to "have something to do," someone came up with the idea of a "school march."

This event usually occurred on the last day (in December or January) at a country school. People came from nearby communities and participated.

A teacher at the host school laid out a route, surrounding the mud, beginning at the schoolhouse. Pupils chose partners of the opposite sex with whom to march. Grownups made their choices. Led by musicians, couples walked about a mile and then retraced their steps.

A friend tells of taking part in such a march. "Miss Polly, our spinister teacher, was in high gear getting everything organized for the march. She accidentally fell backward over a stump. Her long dress went up to her knees. Though unhurt that act took the steam out of Miss Polly. It ruined her day.

"Smiley, the banjo picker, chose his partner. Luby, the gray-haired fiddler, whose wife had recently died (her tracks were still in the yard), asked a pretty young lass for the honor. She turned him down flat. Friends suggested another choice for the fiddler.

"'No!' Luby said curtly, 'If I can't be the tablecloth I won't be the dishrag.'"

Education Then and Now: Some Observations and Opinions

However impossible it might seem for one elementary teacher to instruct a large enrollment in all eight grades, the results speak eloquently.

Teachers at Oil Valley school taught the basics. There were no frills. Also emphasized were social graces and respect for law, the elderly, and for anyone in authority. The children were **disciplined.** Schools turned out citizens, not criminals.

Under this plan the genius of our people blossomed. Creative minds achieved unprecedented breakthroughs in science and the arts. Our nation became the greatest industrialized nation in history. This method cost the taxpayer a fraction of present-day costs.

As a product of this arrangement, I praise it—though I do not impose it. What I do advocate is a return to the **basics** and to **discipline**. Individuality, a time to listen to our own drummer, can come later.

From the Oil Valley school came ministers, farmers, judges, engineers, homemakers, county officers, soldiers, petroleum workers, lumber men, scientists, pharmacists, secretaries, legislators, educators, and one physician, Mack Roberts.

It is wonderful that the time has finally arrived when the attainment of higher education is accessible to all.

However, according to the lament from colleges and universities, too many students arrive ill-prepared. Due to the deterioration of primary and secondary schools, the average score on Scholastic Aptitude Tests fell fifty-six points between 1966 and 1994.

It turns out that too many students cannot spell, cannot calculate, cannot write and have only a slight knowledge of grammar. It is said that more than half of the high school seniors do not know the basics of history. Surely we can do better.

Perhaps most disturbing is the mania for sports (our idolatry) rather than for education.

True, the Kentucky illiteracy rate in the early part of the 20th century was embarrassing. However, the fault, I think, lay not in the teaching methods but in the lack of **required** school attendance. No teacher can prepare a child who is absent.

I recently came across a letter written in 1906 to my maternal grandfather, L.D. Bell, a teacher. The letter from the Superintendent of Public Instruction exhorted each teacher to:

1. Make your own school a standard
2. Help in organizing cooperative teamwork
3. Push your attendance above 60 percent of the census, if possible

Today's administrators strive for above 90 percent of the census. (At a certain percentage of absence due to flu, etc., when the school would lose too much funding, they call off school for everyone.)

The Community

The Country Roads

To keep county roads in a state of repair, the County Judge appointed an overseer in each community. One of his duties was to send a "warning" to each able-bodied male between the ages of twenty-one to sixty-five, to give six days of free labor annually for road service.

The county furnished the tools and dynamite.

On a designated week the men met to ditch the road. For this they used a pick and shovel. They blasted big rocks. They hauled creek gravel or knapped rocks to fill mud holes. Those who did not comply with the notice could be fined or jailed.

Mack performed his stint a number of years.

The practice was terminated in the 1920's.

Toll Roads

Toll roads preceded our present road system.

Private companies built these thoroughfares and erected tollhouses every five miles on the major roads with one near the city limits.

A long pole barrier that extended from a tollhouse across the road was raised to permit the passing of a vehicle, horse and rider, buggy or loaded wagon. Pedestrians were free.

Charges: (Round trips)
Car   30 cents
Buggy   20 cents
Loaded Wagon   40 cents
Horse and rider   10 cents

Travelers were not charged on Sundays, holidays, nor for going to school or church.

Money collected paid for the construction and maintenance of roads.

Stagecoach 1895 - 1915

When Mack was five years old, he traveled with his father to Mill Springs to visit his Uncle Bolen. On this trip he got his first look at our stagecoach.

The red coach made a daily run of twenty miles to the railroad station at Burnside in Pulaski County, carrying mail and passengers. Four fine trotting horses pulled the vehicle.

Stops were made at post offices and tollgates. The coach accommodated nine passengers inside and five passengers on top plus the driver. Baggage traveled on top in the rear. The fare was $1.50 each way. The trip required three to five hours depending on road conditions and the weather. Horses were changed midway at Frazer.

On the hot August day that Mack met the coach with its capacity load, black passengers rode inside the coach, and white travelers sat on top of the vehicle where they could get the breeze—and full sun!

This was the same snazzy coach and four that brought oilmen and other personages to town where they got off at the Ramsey Hotel.

Mr. Charlie Burton owned the stagecoach. In order to have no competition carrying passengers on his mail route, Mr. Burton had bid off the mail route for four years for four cents. Mr. John Huffman usually did the driving of the coach for Mr. Burton.

Gardens

Most everyone in the community had a vegetable garden. If they didn't, they were looked down on.

After plowing and preparing the soil, the men turned the garden over to their wives and daughters. The women took pride in their garden, staking the rows straight, and they tried to keep the garden weed-free. Bugs were not a problem in the early part of the century.

Mack says, "Many of our neighbors planted "according to the moon (zodiac signs). We just planted—when the soil was right and at a convenient time. Mama did insist that we plant our beans on Good Friday."

A rivalry existed in the neighborhood as to who could brag about reaping the first "mess" of peas, beans, tomatoes or corn.

"We ate out of our garden from early April—green onions, mustard, lettuce, radishes and such—until the last crop in the fall—usually turnips and turnip greens."

The boys often invaded the garden for an onion, cucumber or tomato to eat with a piece of cornbread from the kitchen table.

In addition, the farm children ate from the "Wild Kitchen" surrounding valleys and hillsides through the spring, summer, and fall months: serviceberries, strawberries, blackberries, huckleberries, gooseberries, dewberries, grapes, wild grapes, mulberries, papaws, hickory nuts, walnuts, chestnuts and persimmons.

The Singing School

During the winter or spring months, the singing school teacher appeared in the community to teach or reteach the rudiments of music.

The singing master is usually from "away from here." He charges a fee of perhaps a dollar or a dollar and a half per student and a family rate of three dollars.

The interested people assemble early. They stand in groups and discuss everything from the sowing of grass to quilt making.

The teacher already has his black cloth chart stretched across the front of the church or school building. The basic elements of music are on the chart—the chromatic scale, rests, musical terms, time, etc. A red-tipped pointer and tuning fork complete his equipment.

Singers are divided into four groups: soprano, alto, tenor and bass.

The song book has shaped notes: Do, re, me, fa, sol, la, ti, do.

First, the participants learn to sing the **music** of the song. This may be repeated several times with the teacher aiding whichever group that falters.

After the notes are learned well enough to please the enthusiastic teacher, he raps his tuning fork, a small two-pronged instrument, on a table, holds it to his ear and listens to its perfect pitch. The teacher sings, "Do, me, sol, do, sol - mi - do - mi" in measured tones and he's off—leading the song and waving hands in accurate time with the precision of a metronome.

All voices, all harmonizing parts, chime in; discords are drowned by the high sopranos and tenors.

No singing school would be complete without learning a few songs written in the minor key. Mack mentions one such song, *I Will Arise and Go to Jesus*.

Singing schools usually continued for two weeks. They were greatly enjoyed—a social event.

Among the early imported singing school teachers were a Mr. Grimsley, a Mr. Rexroat and Jim E. Floyd.

Mack tells of a neighbor who attended a singing school who said, "I'm not very good on the music (notes), but when it comes to the words, I can sure make 'em howl."

Chautauqua

For a number of years the Chautauqua paid an annual visit to Monticello.

The cultural event took its name from the New York town where it originated in 1874.

This traveling troupe usually came in the summer and presented educational materials and entertainment in a portable tent. The Chautauqua drew large crowds.

Mack tells of one wide-eyed country bumpkin, who, enthralled by the magical moving film, called out, "Ernie, watch that old buzzard [ostrich] lope!"

Haig's Mighty Circus

Though tame by present day standards, a highlight of the year was the annual circus. The big top usually had an elephant or two, caged wild animals and horses with daring riders.

"As kids," Mack says, "we enjoyed the peanuts and Cracker Jack vendors.

"The gravity-defying, tightrope walk highlighted the circus; it set the nerves on edge.

"It was our first introduction to the world of the circus and for many people the only show they ever saw."

Weddings

During this era, weddings in the rural areas were simple family affairs.

Elopement became the alternative and usually occurred for one of three reasons: an underage bride (Kentucky law stipulated the lower limit as age eighteen for the bride), family disapproval, or the romantic excitement of stealing the bride and "running away."

Many couples from Mack's area went to a nearby Tennessee town—Huntsville, Byrdstown, or Jamestown–where they found the law less stringent.

Couples usually traveled by horseback in the earlier years. Mack tells of one fellow who fled with the bride-to-be riding behind him on his horse. As they traveled up a hill the saddle girth broke and both fell off the horse.

Following the wedding, the newlyweds are honored with the "infare," a sumptuous feast at the groom's parents' home. Both friends and families are invited. Mack tells of one such supper where whiskey flowed freely. Some of the male guests stirred their coffee with their pistols.

On their wedding night, the honeymooners could expect the *charivari*—a noisy celebration with kettles, horns, etc.—by their friends and neighbors. The groom might be given a "ride on a fence rail."

The bridal pair lived with one set of parents, usually the groom's, for months or years before they struck it out on their own: children and even grandchildren were born into that home. Many couples spent their lifetime in the groom's parents' home.

If disharmony prevailed, the couple might move out into the nearby two-room "pouting" or "weaning" house built for family newlyweds.

Church

Church, though not a social event, was in a sense a social affair in rural areas in the early decades of the twentieth century.

Because of the lack of transportation, people had few chances to get together. There were those who attended church to worship; others came to see or be seen.

In Mack's earliest years there was no church building in his community, no regular assembling to worship.

However, worship services were sometimes conducted by different denominations in the school building.

"The first time I remember going to church," Mack says, "I rode behind my father on a horse to Big Springs Baptist Church at Burfield, a distance of five miles across the mountain. I must have been about three years old.

"My grandfather Jackson had been partly responsible for building that church. My father had worked on it during its construction.

"While at church, I saw a little girl with dark spiral curls.She wore a green dress. I thought she was the prettiest girl I had ever seen.

"A Bro. Fairchild was the pastor. I remember Luther Barrier was the song leader."

In 1912, the Elk Spring Valley Baptist Church was built near the Oil Valley schoolhouse. The Robertses then worshiped there. Mack later became a member of that congregation.

Mack says, "The brethren sat on the left side and the sisters sat on the right side of the one-room white frame building.

"Mr. John Dodson, father of the Chinese missionary, Miss Flora Dodson, gave the new church a pedal organ. Mrs. T.J. Oatts gave us a hanging oil lamp.

"During the winter months a potbellied stove heated the building.

Throughout the year a preacher came monthly and preached on Saturday mornings, Saturday nights and Sunday mornings

"Families arrived at church by a wagon or on horseback. Teenagers liked to walk. Horses hitched to nearby cedar trees stomped and swished flies with their tails until services were over.

"Church leaders and visiting ministers sat in the 'Amen corner' on the preacher's right.

"'Amens' signaling approval of what the speaker had said were vocal and loud. Many worshipers knelt to pray.

"A water bucket with dipper sat on the pulpit. It was not uncommon for someone, particularly a mother, to bring her baby or brood up front and give them water out of the common dipper during the service.

"The pedal organ squeaked loudly.

"We passed a hat to take up a collection for the preacher. Pastors received little money; times were hard."

Mack's uncle, Reuben Roberts, was pastor of the Shiloh Baptist Church in the 1920s or 30s. Once a month he rode his horse the fifteen mile distance from his home and preached on Saturday morning, Saturday night and Sunday morning. One member of the church gave him fifty cents once—his sole monetary reward.

Dr. C.B. Rankin related that Uncle Billy Cooper, a local well-known Baptist preacher in the latter part of the 19th century, had preached a long time at the same church and had not received **any** compensation.

One Sunday the preacher said, "I've preached here for fifty years, and you never gave me a nickel, and I never asked for a nickel. Now I want $50 so I can go visit my brother in Texas." Dr. Rankin was sure the preacher didn't receive a penny more than the requested amount.

Annual "revivals," always conducted in warm weather, continued for two weeks with both morning and evening services. The entire community turned out to attend. The children from the nearby school attended morning services. Many times, they were asked to recite Bible verses.

Mack says, "A 'fire and brimstone' preacher would start his sermon in a moderate, audible tone of voice and speak for ten or fifteen minutes. Suddenly, he would go into **overdrive**— speaking loudly and rapidly. No one could understand what he said. This would continue for thirty or forty minutes.

"The speaker would return to a normal tone of voice abruptly. This woke the babies and sleeping adults.

"Once a preacher of that type asked my brother, Ottis, how he had liked his sermon.

"'For the first fifteen minutes,' Ottis said, 'I could follow you and thought you were going to preach a good sermon. But when you started selling tobacco I lost all track of what you were saying.'"

On one occasion when church people testified as to "what the good Lord had done for them," a brother asked Caleb to tell what He had done for him.

"He pert nigh ruint me," the freckle-faced, harelipped boy answered.

Preachers never lacked invitations to dinner. They were often served the "gospel bird" (chicken).

A tale is told of an incident that happened in the backwoods of our county. The local church had a history of disruptive behavior during revivals. In fact, in recent years, each preacher who had made an attempt to reach the sinners had been run off.

Many of the neighbors were engaged in making moonshine or delighted in drinking the noxious stuff. The preaching of the word of God had a negative effect on the liquor business.

One dedicated, prominent preacher resolved to try to bring about a change.

News spread of an upcoming gospel meeting.

People had assembled. Among the welcoming committee for the evangelist was a "shiner." He had sat on the doorstep of the church and cradled a half gallon jar of his product in his arms.

During his opening remarks, the preacher said, "I've received a call to hold a revival at this place. I understand hitherto you've been unable to have a meeting here." The minister stood tall, looked at his audience directly and announced loudly, "We will have this meeting." At that point he pulled out of his pocket a .38 revolver and laid it beside his Bible on the stand. The speaker added further, "I just hope I don't have to kill anyone."

It was reported that they had one of the most successful revivals in the church's history.

The Kitchen

As in many households of the period, the Roberts family had grandmother, mother, aunts, and often daughters-in-law ready to prepare the necessary victuals for so many people.

The "cooks" wore their multipurpose aprons. The aprons not only protected clothing during meal preparation, but they were used to carry garden produce, eggs, and chips to start a fire in the Home Comfort cook stove, or to wipe the tears or nose of a crying "young 'un."

Saturdays were spent in dusting the parlor and food preparation for Sunday guests.

Egg beaters twirl, spoons clatter, lard sizzles and pops. The kitchen smells of cloves, allspice, cinnamon and nutmeg.

"Aunt Hannah had a knack for making light bread," Mack says. "Mama made egg custards, gingerbread, stacked pies and tea cakes. Aunt Lytha fried good chicken. Sometimes they made hominy. Other foods were potato salad and eggs pickled in beet juice. The women worked as a team. They defied the saying: "You can't have two queens in one hive."

A single dessert never reigned on the table. Nor were any made from mixes by using electrical appliances. Beating a cake became laborious.

The cooks used few "receipts." Someone might be told to use a pinch of salt or a "glug" of vinegar—or "as much butter as you can afford."

One great-aunt gave out instructions for making pork sausage. "Add your sage and salt and a left handful of red pepper."

The fresh butter, cream and milk in the spring house, the cured hams, bacon and shoulder in the smokehouse, the cackle-fresh eggs, free-range chickens, turkeys and quail, plus the just-picked fruit and top-quality vegetables available would trigger the envy of a French chef.

"Just thinking about those good country meals makes my mouth water," Mack says.

Lazy Susan

Mack says, "My grandfather had a custom-crafted Lazy Susan table." A Lazy Susan was a revolving tray placed at the center of a dining table from which one can help oneself to food.

This table proved to be a valuable asset for such a large family since they had so many guests and the usual quota of "work hands."

Mack tells that one laborer was too shy to turn the table, "but when another diner rotated it, he grabbed a dish as it passed by."

Hospitality abounded in those days.

"We always expected company on County Court Day," Mack says. "Acquaintances on their way to town from Rock Creek, Parmleysville, Kidd's Crossing and Burfield, stopped over for the night with us. I remember one night we had twelve visitors. Grandpap turned our horses out of the barn and stabled the horses of our guests."

Court Day, always on Monday, was a major event. Cases were tried in court and wills probated. Sidewalk salesmen filled their pockets by selling patent medicines and gimmicks. Mule and horse swapping dominated the day.

Activities at Home

Christmas at the Robertses' home was, of course, a family time. They didn't have a Christmas tree. The Christmas tree was at the schoolhouse.

The children hung their stockings by the fireplace and received candy and oranges, cap pistols, firecrackers, Roman candles and such. They celebrated Christmas, rather than the Fourth of July, with fireworks. Their joy surpassed that of a present day child who receives one hundred times as much.

Mack says, "We played outside on Christmas morning until we froze out then made a beeline for the house. We stomped into the warm, steamy kitchen that was fragrant with the smells of roasting turkey, baked fresh ham, vegetables and the spicy aroma of desserts.

"Spoons clattered, the teakettle hissed, conversation hummed and always there was laughter. The Robertses were a jolly family.

"The fragrance of the freshly baked light bread meant the Christmas feast was rising to a crescendo. We could hardly wait to eat.

"Desserts were plentiful: apple stack cake, egg custard with freshly grated nutmeg, sweetbread, gingersnap, dried apple pies, etc. My father used to eat his dessert first so he'd be sure to have room for it.

"In the 1920s it was customary to get the other person's 'Christmas Eve gift and Christmas gift.' We'd wake up soon after midnight on Christmas Eve and Christmas Day and call out 'Christmas Eve gift' or 'Christmas Gift' to everyone." This supposedly obligated the persons to hand over gifts.

Mack tells of a neighbor who arrived in a snowstorm one Christmas Eve. "He stamped his feet on the porch and when we opened the door he hailed us with 'Christmas Ease gift.' He mispronounced 'Eve!' He further added, 'It's snowing so hard you can't see your hand in front of you as far as from here to the gate.'"

After Christmas dinner (at noon) the boys shoot a few rounds of firecrackers, play with their sparklers, then go on their safari.

They return from hunting in time to help with feeding and milking. "By then," Mack says, "that lonesome, after-Christmas feeling set in—the loneliest in the world."

Christmas used to be a time of carousing for many. Some people celebrated Christmas by shooting anvils. They transported the anvils to a high elevation, usually a hilltop, placed one anvil on the ground and filled the opening in the anvil with gunpowder. They set the other anvil on top and lighted a fuse. This caused a deafening sound heard for miles.

Until well into the twentieth century, Old Christmas or Epiphany, which comes on January 6th, had a special meaning to our Appalachian grandparents. By that time, the short days of winter were said to "lengthen a cock's stride" from Christmas to Old Christmas. The cattle in the barn supposedly knelt down in their stalls precisely at midnight on Old Christmas Eve to adore the newborn Babe.

Mack says, "I remember seeing Grandpap Jackson go outside the house on Old Christmas and observe which way the smoke from the chimney blew." Supposedly the weather on Old Christmas and the next eleven days would provide a forecast of the twelve months ahead.

The Robertses Build a New House

In 1916 O.C. Bell and Jim Floyd built the Rhodes Roberts family a new house. Their bill for labor was $180. The chimney and roof were extra.

The two-story frame house, located considerably below the log house, was farther from the spring. The remodeled house is now occupied by Lisle and Ruth Roberts.

Later, Rhodes Roberts acquired adjoining tracts of land until he possessed approximately 1,000 acres—much of it timbered.

Sorghum Making

The Roberts boys were kept home from school to help with the sorghum making.

Every farmer raised a patch of sugar cane. At the right time in the fall, they stripped the cane of foliage, cut it and fed it into a mule-powered grinder that extracted the sweet juice from the stalks.

The community sorghum maker came at the appointed time to make the sorghum. The juice was converted into a thick syrup by boiling it to the right stage in an evaporator. This required close supervision. During the process, the boiling liquid was skimmed of foam and impurities.

No thermometer was required by the experienced sorghum maker to determine when the product was ready. The sorghum was then strained into lard stands or other large containers.

In the meantime, the kids and teenagers chewed on stalks of cane or tried to push one another into the "soup hole" where the "skimmings" had been emptied.

The payoff came the next morning at breakfast when the good stuff was served with hot biscuits, butter, bacon, coffee, etc.

A neighbor counted the number of biscuits eaten one morning by the sorghum maker: 16 huge biscuits, each slathered with a hunk of butter, and eaten with the new "lasses."

Dr. C. B. Rankin kidded, "If a cat can walk across the molasses in cold weather, the molasses is just right."

Mack says, "Sorghum, honey, homemade jellies and preserves provided most of the sweets consumed by a household."

Butchering

Sunshiny days followed by frosty nights make the ideal time for butchering on the farm.

The Robertses usually slaughtered seven or eight hogs, each weighing from 250-500 pounds, every winter. The hogs had been kept in the "fattening pen" for a few months where they gorged on corn, pumpkins and "slop"—that sweet-smelling ambrosia made from kitchen scraps.

Hog killing was a day for neighbors to help one another. Their reward was a big dinner and a "mess of fresh meat" to take home with them.

Ham and shoulders were trimmed of extra fat. This fat was rendered into lard over a hot fire, a long tedious task. The liquid shortening was squeezed from the cooked pieces of pork and strained into a lard stand.

Large families often used seven or eight stands of lard a year. Butter was the only other shortening available. They had never heard of margarine, corn oil or olive oil.

Some leftover pieces of pork (cracklings) from the lard making were often used to make "crackling cornbread"—the best bread in the world if one didn't eat too much!

Hams, middlings and shoulders were cured by treating them with sugar, salt, pepper, and saltpeter. They were then stored in the smokehouse.

Sausage, made from the trimmed shoulders, etc., was canned or stuffed into clean shuck casings.

Everything about the hog but the "squeal" was used. Hogs' heads were made into souse. Pigs' feet were considered a delicacy by many. Brains were mixed with eggs and scrambled. Kids roasted the pigs' tails.

Innocents Abroad

When Mack was sixteen and still in grade school, the Monticello Banking Company and Citizens National Bank gave a Duroc gilt (a young female pig) to each Boy's Club member who wanted one. (The club was forerunner of our present 4-H Club). That was our way of getting a good breed of hogs into the county.

In return for the gilt, the members were required to give the banks two pigs from the first litter.

The banks also awarded a free trip to the State Fair at Louisville, Kentucky, to the one who kept the best record book on the pig project. Mack won the prize.

He had never been out of the county. His world had extended to Burfield on the east and to Cooper on the west and to Mill Springs on the north, a distance of seventeen miles.

His father hesitated to let him go. He knew Mack was inexperienced. He had read earlier of a boy from the mountains of eastern Kentucky who had won a trip to the city. His hotel room had been lighted by an open flame gas light. The boy had been used to extinguishing kerosene lamps by blowing them out. Evidently, he had blown out the gas flame. He was found asphyxiated.

Mack got to make the trip.

He rode to Burnside with the county agent, Mr. Amburgy, and a Boy's Club member from Clinton County. They were to catch the train to Louisville. Mack had never seen a train.

Just when they arrived at Burnside, they heard a 'too-too-too-too-toot' and saw a puffing train—smoke boiling out of the smokestack—enter a tunnel. Seized with fear, Mack just knew they had missed their train. Mr. Amburgy, however, did not appear disturbed.

In a few seconds, the train emerged from the tunnel and hurried northwest, whistling as it went.

They connected with their train later. After an 'All Aboard' their car lurched forward. The car behind rammed them. Again no one seemed alarmed. At last, they were on their way.

They picked up speed, and Mack still remembers the awe of passing through King's Mountain Tunnel. The coal smoke almost suffocated them. He certainly felt good when he again came forth into the daylight.

They switched from the Southern Railway to the L&N Railway at Junction City. They arrived in Louisville at 10:30 p.m. Street cars had stopped running to the fairground.

The county agent got them a couple of rooms at the Capital Hotel on Market Street. However, others shared their rooms.

That night Mack wrote a card home, "I like the country fine," he told his family. They never ceased to tease him about that statement. They had arrived in Louisville after dark.

The next morning they were awakened when someone came through the hall ringing the hand bell. "Five o'clock," he called.

That morning they rode a street car to the state fairgrounds. Mack felt a great distance from home. He thought if the world was as big in the other directions, it was a whopper.

He mailed his postal card at a little post office on the fairgrounds. The man working in the post office wore a button on his coat lapel that said, "To hell with the Kaiser."

They slept in World War I tents next to the poultry and dog

pavilions. The September night was cold and foggy. Even though they used newspapers on their cots for insulation, they nearly froze to death. (They had been instructed to bring a sheet and toothbrush.)

The dogs barked until 2:00 a.m. and then the roosters took over.

The boys had been given tickets to all the shows and exhibits, but they had to pay for their own food. Mack almost got sick on fish sandwiches—ten cents each.

While at the fair, the young fellows were privileged to hear the popular evangelist, Billy Sunday.

They were taken down to the Ohio River to see a big fish on a boat—a manatee. The fish weighed several tons and was 20 feet long.

The officials told them they thought that because it had a bigger throat, this type of fish, rather than a whale, had swallowed Jonah.

Another impressive sight was the Budweiser Beer Wagon. The six horses that pulled the wagon wore fancy harnesses and plumes on their heads that nodded to the beat of their movement.

Mack also saw his first airplane.

On a later trip to the State Fair, Mack and Robert and Ed Dodson attended as Wayne County's livestock judging team. They placed second in the state.

They traveled by Model T with the county agent, Mr. H. J. Hayes, Mr. O. C. Eads and Mr. William West.

"It had rained," Mack says. "We had traveled at breakneck speed of twenty-five miles per hour. Our car chugged and bounced and spit until we came to a hill. Then we'd pile out of the car and push the car up every muddy incline.

"On our way home," Mack says, "we came by Frankfort.

One of the men we traveled with had a neighbor in the penitentiary whom he wanted to visit. We boys went into the prison, too. I remember how dark and narrow the cells were. That was another experience for us."

Mack mentions another trip to the State Fair with Arnold Ramsey and Alfred Shearer. "We traveled by train. One of the fellows had put his train ticket in his hat band. When he opened the window, his ticket blew out. He had to buy another ticket!"

World War I:

The War to End All Wars
and the Post-war Period

The outstanding event of the second decade of the twentieth century was World War I.

During Mack's grade school years, the United States entered the war that had been raging in Europe for three years.

For two and a half years, President Wilson had steadfastly held to his neutral policy. That course changed with the sinking of American ships by Germany. President Wilson then declared it our duty "to make the world safe for democracy; to kill to end killing."

All American men from age eighteen to forty-five were required to register for conscription.

Though unprepared, we entered the war.

In June 1917 our troops landed in France, more than a half a million strong. By October they were in combat.

The number of Americans drafted into the armed forces was 4,800,000. Women served as nurses in the American Expeditionary Force (A.E.F.) and with the Red Cross.

Millions of our men served in the A.E.F. under General John J. Pershing. "Lafayette, we are here," they said at the grave of the Frenchman who came to our aid in the American Revolution.

Mustard gas and other chemical weapons killed or injured thousands of American soldiers in the war.

Though the fighting itself took a great toll—35,000 casualties—winter warfare, in which thousands of soldiers died from influenza and pneumonia, caused ten times as many deaths.

During the war, President Wilson appointed Herbert C. Hoover head of Food Administration. He championed programs to produce and conserve food. Among these were "meatless Tuesdays" and "wheatless Wednesdays."

Mack recalls how that "Kaiser" (Wilhelm), the German ruler, was a despicable name on the tongue of every school child.

War news filtered slowly to the home folk. They heard their news mainly over the telephone party line.

The Robertses had felt the real anxiety of war when Hobart was conscripted and called for a physical examination.

Following the collapse of Germany, the Armistice had been signed in the Hall of Mirrors at Versailles, France, on the eleventh hour of the eleventh day in the eleventh month of 1918. Thankfully this saved Hobart from expected service.

The Allies had lost less than the Central Powers, but a lasting peace was not fashioned.

Later, Mack remembers attending the Veterans Day Parade of the survivors—those who had come home from "over there."

Milestones: The Roaring Twenties

The Roaring Twenties brought great social change.

In 1921, Warren G. Harding succeeded President Wilson, who had become incapacitated while in office.

The most devastating war the world had ever known was over. Society, though, would never be the same.

In 1920 women **won** the right to vote. It is a bit degrading when we realize our nation was a century and a half old before this freedom was gained.

This freedom plus the war years had brought about somewhat of an emancipation for women. They began to work outside the home, bobbed their hair, drank and puffed cigarettes. They wore "flapper" fashions above-the-knee dresses and cloche hats. The Charleston dance became the rage.

In 1923 President Harding died in office and Calvin Coolidge became President. For the first time, radio carried his presidential message to Congress.

In 1923 sedans had become more popular than open cars. Few but the monied could afford cars until the late twenties, when they began to replace horses, wagons, and carriages. The railroad was the main carrier.

By 1923, twenty-three million automobiles hit our highways. This brought about a change in our landscape. Now good roads became a necessity. Filling stations sprang up like morning glories after rain. Billboards advertised everything from "See Rock City" to Lydia Pinkham "Tonic for Women." Burma Shave Verses, strung out on fence posts, entertained.

> *We know*
> How much
> You love that gal
> But use both hands
> For driving pal.
> Use Burma Shave

The auto camping craze began. Tourists courts offered overnight accommodations. An automobile excursion in those days would have been incomplete without a number of punctures. That necessitated jacking up the car, removing the tire, patching the innertube and replacing the tire.

In 1925 John Scopes' "Monkey Trial" tested the validity of teaching evolution. Scopes was convicted then acquitted on a technicality.

In 1927 Charles Lindbergh made the first solo transatlantic nonstop flight.

Hollywood blossomed. Stars of silent pictures received six-figure salaries. Among the famous were Mary Pickford—American Sweetheart—and her husband, Douglas Fairbanks. Others were Rudolph Valentino, Charlie Chaplin, Greta Garbo, Clara Bow, Al Jolson and Walt Disney's Mickey Mouse. Movies were required to show "Compensating values" (the bad guy lost in the end).

The big change came when sound came to the movies in 1927. Radio took over. We were all ears. Radio broadcasted news, sports, entertainment, and commercials. Following WWI our country appeared prosperous. Factories hummed and jobs were multiplied. Model T Fords were coming off the assembly line at the rate of one every second.

Skyscrapers transformed the appearance of cities. Profits skyrocketed. However, the tariffs, the prohibition amendment, and other factors had left behind the heavily mortgaged farmers. Many farmers were driven into bankruptcy. By the end of the decade, 1.5 million farmers left for the city seeking greener pastures.

At the same time life for the mill workers proved no better. Long hours and low wages prevailed. It is ironic that in an age of rising fortune and seeming prosperity, credit reverses in agriculture, plus frantic speculation in the stock market brought about the "crash" of 1929.

High School, College and Medical Scool

Mack entered Monticello High School, the only high school in the county, in 1921, at age eighteen. Few people from the county schools attended secondary schools because of lack of transportation.

"During my freshman year," he says, "Ottis, who was a senior, and I drove the eight-mile distance in a buggy drawn by Old Daisy. We left mare and buggy in a cow barn near school, behind Uncle Wolford Vickery's grocery store on College Street.

"For the first semester of the next year, I drove the buggy alone. I remember Uncle Wolford borrowed my horse to ride up on Morris Hill to collect a debt. On the way, Old Daisy dropped dead. Thereafter, I drove Uncle George Orr's car for his daughter, Jewell, who also attended high school.

"The school building stood on College Street.

"At midterm of my second year, the schoolhouse burned. I completed that year of schooling in the First Baptist Church. In my senior year, classes were held in the Methodist Church." Mack completed high school in three years and one summer term.

"We county students didn't receive a royal welcome. Our 'town' classmates regarded us as 'hayseeds,' made snide remarks and bullied us. A smart aleck sat behind me in class. He jabbed and punched me when he got a chance. I endured this for two or three weeks before I decided to see if I could change his attitude.

"One day when I entered the classroom and sat at my desk before the teacher arrived, my antagonist made some remark that I didn't appreciate. I arose and my right fist made a solid connection under his left jaw.

"The fellow seemed to get the idea—no more harassment. We were good friends thereafter.

"We had the usual curriculum, which included two years of Latin." (Mack still conjugates the verb "to love" in Latin.)

Mack reminisces:

"One of my classmates, who later became a professional man, would have never got through high school if the building hadn't burned. We were simply asked how many credits we had. All records had been destroyed.

"Our school had a good basketball team. They got to the State Tournament. The players were Robert Shearer, Andrew York, Bobby Lee, Alfred Shearer, Grider Anderson and Edwin Smith.

"Our Literary Society met twice a month. We also had debates, piano recitals and such.

"Alfred Shearer, Edwin Smith and I were on the program for a song. We went down the street to Dick Burnett's and had him teach us *A Short Life of Trouble*. That was a pretty big hit."

Graduation exercises were held at the First Baptist Church, 1924. Mack remembers the class motto: "Ahoy, the rapids are below you."

He was valedictorian of his class.

Now to find his niche in society...

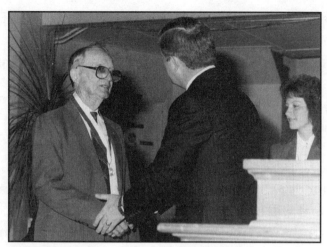

*Dr. Roberts, an inductee into the Alumni Association Hall of
Honor, Cumberland College, Williamsburg, Ky. 1988.*

Cumberland College

"Both of my older brothers had considered attending college but got married instead," Mack says.

"When I graduated from high school, age twenty-one, Dr. O. M. Carter, a family friend and physician, called for me to stop by his office on Columbia Avenue.

"Dr. Carter gave me a fountain pen for a graduation gift and asked me if I'd ever considered studying medicine. I hadn't. He told me that doctors probably lived a little better than the average person, that they could help their fellow man and bring sunshine into the lives of many people." Dear Dr. Carter ignited the dream.

"That put me to thinking about it. I had thought previously about studying engineering. I liked math.

"During our senior year in high school, a representative from Cumberland College, a junior college in Williamsburg, Kentucky, had visited us, soliciting students for the college. It was our nearest college, approximately sixty miles away. I had never heard of the college.

"I applied for admission to the college. I told them I had no money. They asked for me to send my grades.

"I received a letter telling me to 'come on over, we'll take care of you.'

"I had sold my 'bank' pigs and had $44.

"The night before I left for college, my father, who had already gone to bed, asked how much money I had. He said for me to look in the pocket of his pants hanging on the bedpost. He had a two-dollar bill. 'Give me a dollar and you can have the $2; that will make you $45.'

"Early the next morning, my father took me to Monticello in our first car, a Model T, to catch the Wayne County Taxi, driven by Fred Crouch, to Burnside.

"From Burnside I rode the Southern Railway to Junction City. I transferred there to the L&N Railway for Williamsburg.

"I spent twenty-five cents to get my trunk hauled to the boys' dormitory, Felix Hall, at the college.

"They sent me to Mr. Jimmy Ellison, who controlled the McComb College Fund for deserving students.

"I walked past Mr. Ellison's house five or six times before I got up the nerve to knock on his door. He asked me every question in the world until he found out that I was from Monticello. That's where he had met his wife! I obtained a loan that covered tuition, supplies and the $15 a month room and board. The money would be interest free until I was out of school."

Mack still remembers the date he got out of school to go home at Christmas break, December 18. On his return trip to Williamsburg he had a ten-hour layover at Junction City.

During his second year at the junior college, Mack had a job as janitor on the third floor of his dormitory. The job paid $10 a month.

President Creech owned some property near the water tower. He hired Mack and another student to help him do some fencing a few times. He paid 30 cents an hour.

Mack completed his two years at the Baptist college in 1926.

Many years later he was honored as one of the outstanding 100 students of Cumberland College.

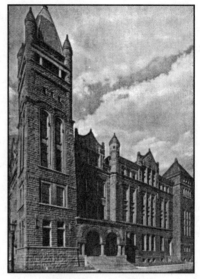

University of Louisville School of Medicine

University of Louisville

Following graduation from Cumberland College in 1926, Mack borrowed money from the Monticello Banking Company and attended the University of Louisville for his premedical requirements.

"The University had no dormitories," Mack says. "Hobart had told me I could stay at the YMCA for $1.50 a night until I could find accommodations. However, I found the YMCA was full!

"I came out of the YMCA and saw the Brown Hotel up the street. I went in and inquired the price of a room.

"'Three dollars and up, Sir'."

"I walked down the street until I came to the Henry Clay Hotel. Their rooms were two dollars. I spent the night there. In the next day or so, I ran into a former Cumberland College classmate who would also attend U of L, Clyde McClure. He lived out at Mt. Washington, twenty miles from Louisville. He asked me to live with his family, and we would commute. I stayed with him the first year."

During the summer term, Mack served as an orderly at the City Hospital. The job paid ten dollars a month, plus board and laundry.

"As an orderly I performed menial tasks: cleaning, making beds, emptying bedpans, answering phones and such.

"I stayed in the Employees Home. I'd wake up on those hot summer nights and kill a dozen bed bugs on the bed.

"The management couldn't get rid of the bed bugs. They would put the mattresses in the autoclave; they would take the iron bedsteads outside and use a blow torch around the crevices. Those bugs must have been in the walls. We had no insecticides nor air-conditioning."

Mack completed his final premedical requirements in a year and one summer term. He received his AB degree after the first year in medical school.

"The next year I **dropped out of school because of lack of funds**. I taught a seven-month school at Dry Fork at Gregory, in Wayne County for seventy-one dollars a month."

"I boarded in the community. We arose early in the morning, had breakfast and then sat around and waited for daylight so we could do the feeding of the livestock.

"I rode a horse back and forth home on weekends.

"One cold Sunday afternoon I was caught in a blizzard as I returned to Dry Fork. Every time I batted my eyes, they froze together.

"I worked at home after the end of the seven-month school term until July of the next year. I then taught two months at Griffin. The next summer I taught two months at Carr School. I returned to Louisville in September to enter the University of Louisville School of Medicine."

Logging

During summer vacations from high school and also college, Mack did some logging. "One year," he says, "we had sold some poplar to the Burnside Veneer Mill. We were to deliver the logs to the Cumberland River at Mill Springs, Kentucky, where they would be picked up by a barge and taken to Burnside." (This was before the Wolf Creek Dam was constructed.)

"We hauled our logs on a wagon pulled by four mules to Mill Springs. The problem was to take them over the narrow steep road to the river.

"One day I started over the hill with 700 or 800 feet of logs. I sat on the saddle mule (left wheeler). My brakes broke; that immediately shot me and my wheelers up into the leaders (the front mules).

"I put the whip to the leaders and got them out in front and finally managed to get the wagon over the upper side of the road. The other side of the road was a steep drop off; tops of trees edged the road.

"I took one chain off the logs and locked a hind wheel and was able to get my load over the hill to the unloading place.

"If my wagon had gone off on the other side of the road, driver, mules, logs and all would have plunged 100 feet.

"I think that was my closest brush with death."

Another summer he hauled lumber out of Crouch Hollow, near Mt. Pisgah, to Oil Valley for Christian Lumber Company.

"I tied my bag lunch to the harness of a mule and left home very early. I furnished four mules and wagon. I returned home after dark. I made seven dollars a day."

Louisville in the 1920s and 1930s

During the years of the Depression, Louisville as well as the nation felt the economic crunch. Everything was cheap, but money was hard to get. Bread sold for a nickel a loaf. Men's shoes sold for $2.85. Men's suits sold for around twenty-four dollars.

There were no expressways, television stations or trucking lines in Louisville.

Model Ts, Chevrolets, and Dodges were the most common cars, though a few prestigious folk drove Franklins, Stutzes or Packard touring cars with isinglass curtains that were snapped into place in bad weather.

Streetcars attached to their overhead umbilical cords rattled their way through the city. Although cars had replaced carriages, there was no bridge except the railway bridge across the Ohio River. One ferry plied the river; it carried as many as thirteen cars per load.

Some fifty trains entered and exited the city daily.

Before suburban sprawl and shopping malls, Fourth Street hummed with traffic, shoppers and theater goers.

Rialto and Loews theaters were in their heyday.

Ladies attired in dress clothing, high heels, hats and gloves, shopped at fragrant Byck's, Selman's or Stewart's Department Store. Then they lunched in the Orchid Room at Stewart's, reached by an elevator manned by a white-coated operator.

Farmers brought their produce to the Haymarket on Market Street.

Vendors pushed ice cream carts through the neighborhood and blew whistles to alert the kids.

The main hotels were the Brown, the Henry Watterson, the Seelbach, the Henry Clay, and the Kentucky.

Belknap Hardware and Bacon Dry Goods were well-known stores.

Mack said, "Early in the morning, before daybreak, we would hear the clopping on the cobblestones of the big old mare that pulled the Ewing Von Allman milk wagon. They left on our doorstep bottles of milk with yellow cream three or four inches deep in the neck of the bottles. They took away the empty bottles left out the night before.

"The Arctic Ice Company had a one-horse wagon pulled by a Belgian horse, that delivered blocks of ice for ice boxes in the homes. Cards specifying the number of pounds wanted were posted in a window. The barber pole still turned. A shave cost ten cents. Haircuts were twenty-five cents. A shoe shine cost five cents."

Signs of the Depression were ever present. Hopes for recovery rested on President Franklin D. Roosevelt. He initiated the "New Deal" and by his dynamic leadership and primarily through his radio "fireside chats," brought about a rebirth of hope for our economy.

University of Louisville Medical School 1928-1932

Mack roomed with J. H. Horton and his wife on 3rd Street during his first year in Medical School. Horton, a Wayne Countian, was also a medical student. Room and board cost thirty-five dollars a month.

Mack was initiated into Theta Kappa Psi, medical fraternity.

The second year he shared an apartment with three other fellow students on Broad Street. They had a hot plate and did some of their own food preparations.

He says, "Certain jobs were available for third and fourth year students. I got a coveted job as student intern at the Emergency Room of City Hospital. For that I received board, room and laundry, plus thirty dollars a month. I worked all night every other night.

"At the City Hospital we took care of the emergencies as they arrived. Saturday nights and holiday nights were terrible. We worked all night, mainly suturing lacerations from the fighting that occurred."

During his junior year, many times he went out in the city by ambulance to help bring in emergency cases. "We drove with the siren wide open, rang the bell, and created quite a stir.

"They sent us out two at a time in the city to deliver babies. An ambulance took us out and turned us loose. One night we didn't get through with the delivery until 2:00 a.m. The streetcars had quit running. We had to walk the two to three mile distance all the way back to the hospital carrying the two heavy bags."

In his senior year he had the same position except it didn't pay the thirty dollars. They were not required to make the ambulance runs as during the previous year.

Mack says, "We had ninety-six in our class—one woman. On the first day of school we heard an address by Dr. Irvin Abell, a nationally known physician; I remember one thing the physician said. 'If you are getting into the field of medicine thinking you will get rich, you've chosen the wrong profession. You should have chosen law. A patient will give a lawyer $5,000 to keep him out of the gates of the penitentiary, when he wouldn't give a doctor $500 to keep him out of the gates of hell!'

"The most alarming news came by the grapevine. Traditionally during the first two years the University flunked out about twenty percent of the students in order to accommodate applicants from southern medical junior colleges.

"Already strapped financially, now we had the fear of failing.

"Beginning on the first day, we devoted each afternoon to cadaver dissection. Two students worked on the upper part of the body, two on the lower part.

"Sometimes this initial introduction to medical school caused students to drop out. That didn't happen in our class.

"Testing time was inhumane. In one class an old German professor stood on top of his desk to make sure of no cheating. 'Keep your heads down—I will throw you out!' he shouted."

Mack still dreams about the brutality of medical school.

"True to the grapevine telegraph, at the end of our school year, twenty members of the class were flunked—some of whom were later admitted to another medical school elsewhere and made a name in the medical profession.

"After the first two years, there was no failing. We still had to study hard, but the pressure was off. The professors were kind and respectful.

"Though I worked all night every other night at the hospital, I carried a full study curriculum. I enjoyed no recreation—work, work, work. I attended one movie during my freshman year."

Mack attended the Walnut Street Baptist Church when not on call. Finley Gibson was the pastor.

Mack vividly remembers one night. "I was hard at work—studying, when about 10:00 p.m., I heard a newspaper boy going down the street calling, 'Extra, extra, Monticello burns down.'

"I rushed out and bought the extra edition of the Louisville *Courier Journal*. It told about the fire that destroyed an entire block on Main Street: Shearer-Eads General Store, Grover Burton's Pool Room, Ramsey Drug Store (owned by Carl Rankin and Kay Huddleston), and Shearer-Casteel Hardware, one of the largest hardwares in the state, handling oil supplies, wagons, buggies, etc.

"The fire also wiped out the well-known Ramsey Hotel across the street.

"The fire occurred during our 22-inch snow of 1929."

After Mack's graduation from medical school, the much-dreaded Medical State Board Examination presented the next hurdle. Mack says, "We didn't shave and hardly ate or slept during that time."

He came through victoriously. At last, he became a licensed physician.

Medical school was not a good memory. He says, "The first two years of medical school were the most miserable, challenging years of my life." Many years later, when we were in Louisville, Mack made it a point to avoid the Old Medical School building.

Now at age 28, he was free of school at last. The preparation had been long and arduous. He had felt the economic pinch all the way.

He persevered in order to qualify for a profession that would deprive him of much social and family life. He would face flood, rain, sleet and snow to minister to those he would serve—and would love it so much he would hardly be able to give it up when he finally retired.

When our grandson, Mark, who was in medical school, prepared for an anatomy test, in a phone conversation his grandfather told him the first question he had had on his **first** practical anatomy test (66 years ago)!

Milestones

In the summer of 1933, Mack traveled to the Windy City for the Chicago World's Fair celebrating "a century of Progress."

Though we were still in the depths of the Depression, the fair drew more than forty million people.

The Great Depression touched everyone. Among those hardest hit were the farmers. Hogs sold for $2.85 a hundred-pound; tobacco sold for three cents a pound; corn ten cents a bushel. Following the greatest drought in history, churning black clouds moved across the Great Plains piling mountains of dust—covering homes, burying livestock, etc. The devastation set off a migration of farm families. Many went to California.

During the time of this economic tragedy, several writers appealed to the reading public with books that identified with their misfortune. Among these writers were William Faulkner, John Steinbeck, Margaret Mitchell and Pearl S. Buck.

Entertainment by radio, during this period of gloom, proved to be the main affordable pursuit.

We listened to soap opera, Edgar Bergen and his dummy, Charlie McCarthy, Glenn Miller and Benny Goodman, Bing Crosby, Kate Smith, Amos 'n Andy.

Crime during the Depression provoked widespread fear. The Lindbergh kidnaping was the crime of the century. John Dillinger succeeded Pretty Boy Floyd as Public Enemy #1. The Federal Bureau of Investigation, headed by J. Edgar Hoover, became a powerful force in dealing with criminals.

Health Officer
1932-1938

With his laborious years behind him, Mack, armed with a medical diploma, was ready to enter the world of medicine. He remained a bachelor, though he had dated a nursing student during those years.

"I had heard," he said, "that Dr. Russell Teague, our local health officer, had applied for a leave-of-absence to further his specialization.

"Before going home from Louisville, I went to see Dr. Phillip Blackerby at the State Board of Health, and applied for the position.

"I got the job. Dr. Teague left in August and I became Wayne County Health Officer. Teague had earned an annual salary of $3,600. Because of the Depression, I received $2,600. My office, over Rankin Drug Store, was provided, but I had to furnish my own car.

"I bought a second-hand Ford Coupe in Louisville for $125. The tires looked pretty good. One day I went on a call to Sunnybrook. The W.P.A. had recently put limestone rocks in the mud holes in the road. Those sharp rocks cut my tires to pieces. When I got home, I had to buy four new tires.

"A former classmate, Miss Elizabeth Parrigin, was already the County Health nurse. She became my helper.

"We emphasized Preventive Medicine. We visited each of the eighty County schools three times during the school year to immunize children against typhoid, diphtheria, whooping cough and smallpox."

Some schools could not be reached by car because of impassable roads. Mack rode a horse to visit many schools. This sometimes necessitated spending the night along the way.

On one such occasion, he went coon hunting with the men folk. The next day before he left, the family asked for a prescription for "the itch"—they all had it, they said. Mack didn't catch the itch!

Other duties included giving physical examinations to school children, conducting prenatal clinics and treating the indigent. Mack delivered a few babies during this time, though that was not among his duties.

Special emphasis was put on the treatment and eradication of venereal disease.

In the meantime, Dr. Teague moved on to a higher position.

Mack paid off his $3,000 debt to the Monticello Banking Company.

He remained a bachelor.

Internship and Private Practice

After Mack's years as Health Officer, he interned for one year (1938-39) at St. Joseph's Hospital in Lexington, Kentucky.

He relates, "It was a nice learning experience. I came in contact with the leading doctors in Lexington. I had the privilege of working with Dr. Fred Rankin, an eminent surgeon, son-in-law of Dr. Charles Mayo. People came to him from all over the United States."

During Mack's internship, his brother Kermit entered the hospital with a staphylococcic septicemia. Antibiotics had not made their appearance, and despite all efforts to save him, Kermit died. He left a wife and four little girls.

The family circle had been broken. His had been the first

death in the family. Kermit was only twenty-nine years old.

Returning home in 1939, still a bachelor, Mack opened his private office.

He and Dr. W. R. Tuttle, a beloved dentist and friend, shared a suite of offices in the Rankin Building on the Square. They used the same waiting room. Mack had no office help during his early years of practice.

After our marriage in 1941, I helped in the office some until our babies came. When our daughters entered college, I worked with Mack again until my father had a stroke.

Thereafter, Aleta Roberts became his faithful helper for twenty-seven years. In the meantime, Jo Ann Powell (Anderson), employed by Dr. Tuttle, served as a wonderful receptionist for Mack.

"Beginning a practice took a little time," he calls to mind. "The economy continued to be bad. People didn't visit the doctor unless they were **sick.** If a patient couldn't get another doctor, he would call me. Office calls were $1.00; house calls in town, $2.50.

"We charged a dollar a mile for calls out in the county. Tonsillectomies were twenty-five dollars. We delivered babies for twenty-five dollars (thirty dollars for twins), regardless of distance, time spent, road conditions, or complications."

Contemporary doctors in Monticello were Dr. C. B. Rankin, Dr. Frank L. Duncan, Dr. Perry Parrigin, Dr. E. B. Rice, Dr. Theopholis Gamblin and Dr. C. F. Holtegel. Dear Dr. O. M. Carter had died during Mack's internship in Lexington.

When Mack entered private practice in our southeastern county of Wayne, three-fourths of our population lived on farms. Only about one-half of the farms could be reached by improved roads.

Eighty-five percent of rural homes had no electricity. Ninety-seven percent had no toilet. Many patients lived below the poverty level.

Our state, at this time, ranked near the bottom of our 48 states in education, particularly in literacy. Fully thirty percent of its adults over twenty-five were illiterate and more than twenty percent of our children didn't attend school.

Tuberculosis was still epidemic, with 14,000 active cases in the state. Dr. C. C. Howard of Glasgow, a champion of rural medicine, pushed the state to build five TB sanitariums.

Several hundred Kentuckians died of typhoid each year. Diphtheria, malaria and whooping cough were rampant; even scarlet fever was widespread.

Pneumonia, that often followed influenza, was a real killer. "We had to treat pneumonia symptomatically," Mack recalls. "We had no antibiotics. We treated the cough and the pain. The fever usually broke on the fifth, seventh, or ninth day. Why on those odd days no one ever figured out."

"Our main drugs were quinine for malaria, digitalis for heart disease, and mandelamine for urinary tract infections."

"Syphilis was treated with shots of bismuth and neo-salvarsan. Aspirin, chloroform, and morphine were used for pain."

Doctors performed their miracles with crude instruments and the help of God.

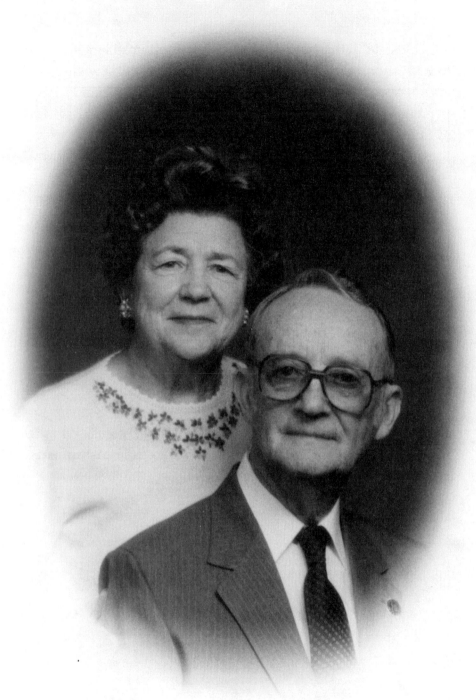

Alma and Mack Roberts, c. 1985

PART II: 1933-2000
We

Marriage, Family, Medical Practice, Retirement

We

Whoever loved that loved not at first sight?
–Christopher Marlowe

The first year I attended Monticello High School (1932) I rode the five-mile distance with four other students from our community, most of whom graduated that year.

The second year presented a transportation problem. Mack was Wayne County Health Officer at that time. His schedule was similar to school hours and he drove past my home.

My father approached Mack about transporting my sister Shirley and me. He kindly agreed to accommodate us.

I doubt that I had ever spoken to Mack. I had simply admired him from afar.

I remember vividly the first time I ever saw him. If my extrasensory perception had been working, I would have realized that day would be unforgettable.

An eighth grader, I'll admit I was at an age to be easily smitten—the tender romantic age of fourteen. On that summer afternoon Oil Valley School had dismissed, and I, along with a classmate, had walked down the hill from the schoolhouse to the road.

We met two young men approaching the school building. One wore white clothing. When they were out of hearing, with admiration in my voice, I asked, "Who is that fellow in white?

He's the best-looking man I ever saw." Of course, I had never seen those Spanish policemen.

Surprised, my friend Leila said, "Don't you know him? He's Mack Roberts, our teacher's brother. He is in medical school."

No, I had had no occasion to meet him: though we lived in the same community, we attended different churches. Our paths had not crossed. Then I recognized an age disparity; I knew not how much.

That summer Mack was home from medical school. One day when he had helped with farm work, I saw him drive a wagonload of wheat past our house.

I had stood mesmerized and watched him for a quarter of a mile, until his wagon turned out of sight.

Now I would be riding to school with him. I immediately turned into a shy person in great awe of Dr. Roberts.

At the end of the year my sister graduated from high school. Two years remained of my high school education.

For the next two years I continued to ride with Mack, along with his brother Harry, who had been an excellent teacher at Oil Valley and was now Wayne County's Attendance Officer.

Riding daily with them, I gradually overcame my timidity. I found Mack to be fun-loving, witty and thoughtful.

For a little girl wearing a wind-blown hairstyle and Tangee lipstick straight from the 5 and 10¢ store, those days were spent in fanciful musings. My heart told me one thing but my mind said, "Ridiculous!"

Mack and I enjoyed some lively debates over politics. He was a Republican and I a Democrat. Franklin Delano Roosevelt had been elected president, and I admired him greatly. Mack and I discussed many things and developed a real camaraderie. Sometimes he took me on calls with him.

For two summers, on Sunday afternoons, Mack and I, along

with Mack's sister Joyce and my sisters Mayme and Shirley, had played croquet with our neighbors, Bryles and Odell Campbell.

Mack and I were croquet partners. "Your mallet had a blue stripe and mine a yellow stripe," he still remembers.

I can see him now as he knelt to help me line up a shot against our opponent. "Now if you don't send him on a journey, young lady, I'll never have anything more to do with you." I tried hard. He had to overlook my poor skill.

Later, one afternoon at the end of my school term, he took me to Lock 21 at Eadsville (before the Wolf Creek Dam was built). I had never been there.

Only a few days ago when we reminisced about that trip he said, "You wore a white dress." Yes, one I had made in my Home Economics class.

Later, while a college student, I accepted his invitation to accompany him on his all-day round to visit some county schools to vaccinate the children.

We picnicked that day in the world's best picnic spot—by a tree-canopied spring that gushed icy water. What a pleasant memory!

I often wondered, does Mack see me as just a giddy kid or does he enjoy my company? Do I see him with my heart or eyes?

Answer: Both! I had found my Prince Charming. That man had captured my heart.

I wished. . . .

I thought Mack had never laid eyes on me until I had become a passenger in his car. "I saw you first," he told me later. "We were walking home from school and met your family moving into our community. You were in your mother's arms."

Between my junior and senior years in high school I made the greatest decision of my life: I became a Christian.

Mack had witnessed my confession that Jesus is the Christ, the Son of the living God. I was baptized into Christ and thus added to His church.

Now that I had graduated from high school (1936), Mack's path and mine would diverge. <u>Paradise lost!</u>

Love's Hope Springs Eternal

"When you wish upon a star;
makes no difference where you are. . . "
– Ned Washington

After graduation from high school my only thought had been the continuance of my education. I sought a teacher's certificate; at that time two years of college met the requirement.

My first year I spent at Cumberland College. The next year I enrolled at Western State Teachers College. I led a busy college life. I studied hard. I dated.

I wondered about the risks of an eligible "bachelor" (that word always intrigued me) at the mercy of women with their feminine wiles. How long would he continue his single life?

Mack had once told me of an infatuated teacher who had written him, "I can't live without you," she had said. (She survived.)

I <u>wished</u> that man shared my fascination. . . .

Whoever said that the path of true love is easy?

I returned home and taught school at Jennings Hollow. The seven-month term extended from July until mid-January. That allowed me to return to college for the second semester and a couple of summer terms.

Those were busy years. I taught for two years with only a weekend between the teaching term and reentering college and vice versa.

Throughout those years that nonstop daydreaming persisted. I waited for that bachelor. I <u>wished</u> I could be near him.

In the meantime, I changed my major from Education to Home Economics. It had been Mack's suggestion.

That act cost me my college degree. To change my major added many more required hours.

When I returned home from college in August 1939, I learned Mack had left for a year's internship at St. Joseph's Hospital in Lexington, Kentucky. Now that I was home, he was away. Our schedules weren't in harmony, to say the least. Disgusting! Anyway, he's still a bachelor, I told myself. In spite of that undertow of hopelessness, I wished. I waited.

There had been little correspondence between us. Was it true that absence makes the heart grow fonder—or fonder of someone else? I would see.

In the summer of 1940, I had completed my last summer term at Western, a memorable year.

My parting words to a young lover had been, "I'm going home and marry Dr. Mack Roberts." In retrospect that had been quite a leap of faith and I hadn't read *The Power of Positive Thinking.* It hadn't been written.

God moves in miraculous ways his wonders to perform. Unbeknown to me, a young doctor who had just completed his internship and had opened his office in Monticello, Kentucky, one hundred miles east of Bowling Green, entertained the same thoughts!

Mack and I were drawn as if by magnets.

No longer a teenager, I returned home and began my third teaching term.

I knew Mack was back home. He had not married or I would have heard.

I wished I could enjoy his company.

Now we were both home. I made no attempt to see him. We did not meet by coincidence.

> *Climb every mountain*
> *Ford every stream*
> *Follow every rainbow*
> *Till you find your dream.*

–Rogers and Hammerstein, *Sound of Music*

Paradise Regained!

*"Think not that you can direct the course of love,
for love,if it finds you worthy, directs your course"*
–Kahil Gibran

Strangely enough, dreams carried around in our hearts for years have a way of abruptly materializing.

With the coming of the autumn season had come the ripening of affection.

Then came a glorious day in October, 1940. I wonder why I didn't wake that morning with a prescience that it would be a red-letter day?

Some moments in life though are just too sacred to divulge. These are our own secrets, shared only with that full moon.

Suffice it to say that Mack and I were together that enchanted evening—actually by happenstance on my part, but by design on Mack's. He knew where to find me!

It had been a Helen Hunt Jackson "bright blue weather" type of October day.

Now, the kaleidoscope of the turning leaves had softly melted into dusk. A cool breeze, soft as eiderdown, carrying the pungent scent of burning leaves, swayed thin-leafed branches and whispered winter would come.

In a star-studded sky, the fat moon paused long enough to wink and furnish its magic to that couple on that special reunion occasion.

Diamonds twinkled in the heavens, love sparkled in our hearts. We didn't discuss the weather.

We agreed that nine years of waiting was long enough. We decided to live our lives together forever happily—married, of course. For two cautious individuals it didn't take us long to make that decision. We hadn't even consulted a marriage counselor!

We planned to marry at the end of my teaching term—within three months. Furthermore, we decided to keep our plans secret until the date drew near. Then we would tell our families.

Paradise Regained!

Now we had nine years to make up.

Bob Wills and His Boys struck up "Beer Barrel Polka" on the car radio, keeping rhythm with my heart.

Hadn't Elizabeth Barrett Browning said, "Every wish is like a prayer to God"? Henceforth I must be very careful about my wishes; they had a way of coming true.

Now to home and sweet dreams. Intoxicated with happiness, I went to sleep at 4:45 A.M. That morning I woke to love at first light. Ah, sweet mystery of life, at last I'd found it!

Sweet Remembrance

*"The entire sum of existence is the magic of being
needed by just one person."*
–Vic Putnam

I smile when I remember how many times, as a child, I had
told my fortune by plucking the petals from a daisy as I sat flat
on the ground and made a daisy chain. "He loves me, he loves
me not, he loves me, he loves me not"—yes, he loves me!

Rich man
Poor man
Beggarman, Thief
<u>Doctor</u>, Lawyer
Merchant, Chief

Now, however, I was old enough to know if I married a doctor I would play second fiddle to his profession. But I didn't
realize I would sometimes play <u>bass</u>!

I tried to analyze my elation. Like Adam I had fallen in love
at first sight; but I had taken a second look.

My love was not based on Mack's handsomeness, though
that didn't hurt any. True, that had been the initial attraction.

He was of average height and well-built. He had broad shoulders and perfect posture; he walked tall.

My friend had dark brown hair, a high forehead, blue eyes, a
beautiful nose and a cleft chin. I liked his heavy dark beard—always
there was a four o'clock shadow. He radiated a glow of humor.

Hadn't my mother warned her daughters, "Not all is gold that glitters"? Right!

My interest had been instantaneous, but Mack was everything I admired in a man, and we had the same moral values. He represented maturity, intelligence, and tranquility, and he seemed to need me.

"I say he's too old for you," my spinster aunt had said. It suited my pride that he was older than I. Furthermore we had affinity of the soul, mind and spirit. What he saw in me I had no idea. Love is blind, they say, and I am glad.

Dr. Samuel Johnson said, "An unmarried man is only half a man." I would make that man whole!

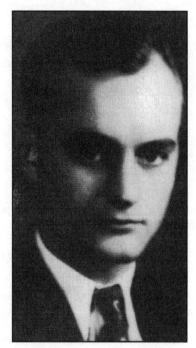

Wm. R. Tuttle, D.D.S.,
a dear friend who shared a
reception room with Dr. Roberts
throughout his career.

Never had I treasured privacy so much. I liked being alone—listening to the song of my own thoughts. I went around as if in a trance.

Now that Mack had established himself in his office, he lived at the Cooper Hotel.

I, along with three other teachers, rode a school bus to our respective county schools.

Mack arose early each morning and came down to the Rankin Drugstore and watched me leave for school from the Silver Star Restaurant. In the afternoons, he sometimes took me home.

We dated mainly on weekends. We attended movies, or he

came to my home, and I often accompanied him on calls.

We didn't have many plans to finalize. Neither of us, quiet individuals that we are, would consider anything but a private marriage ceremony.

After marriage, I would share his room at the hotel until we could find an apartment and buy our furniture.

We talked and talked.

Religion? I had my own convictions, he had his faith: Baptist. I, as a member of the Church of Christ, would remain there. What about the children, if any? They would make their own decisions.

I did innocently stipulate that I would accompany Mack on his night calls as well as the calls he made during the daytime.

I soon got a taste of what life would be married to a doctor. He "stood me up" several times while we dated when he got a call after we had made plans. But he always called to tell me.

Sometimes at night I heard him "toot" when he passed our house, going or returning from I knew not where, and on occasions when I had not heard him, my mother had!

Believe it or not, I got my first inkling of patient interference in our lives when they came to <u>my home</u> for Mack when he was there on a date!

Mack found our dog, Sport, to be a formidable foe. Every time Mack approached the door, Sport went into a fit of growling and barking and jumped at him when he entered.

Mack added to Sport's fury by flipping gravels at him. He also accused the family of training the dog. In all the thousands of house calls the doctor made, Sport was the only dog he couldn't win.

I cannot say time passed quickly. Those winter days, though short, were long to me. January finally arrived. On the morning of our wedding day, Mack, while in the Rankin Drugstore, had remarked to his dear pharmacist friend, Carl Rankin, "If I had a new hat, I'd get married." "I'll furnish the hat," Carl said. Together they went across the street to Bill Wray's Clothing Store, where Carl purchased the hat.

Another dear friend, dentist Dr. W. R. Tuttle, accompanied them to the store.

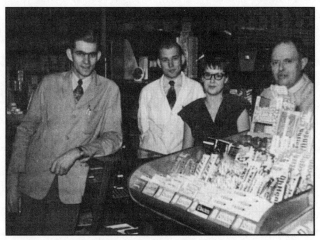

The staff at Rankin Drug Store, 1951
(left to right) Howard Smith, Alvin Bertram,
Maxine Ogden; and Carl Rankin,
pharmacist, owner and dear friend.

God's Grace

"And we know that all things work together for good to them that love the Lord."
–Romans 8:28

It makes me shudder to think of what might have happened during those intervening years.

"I waited until you grew up," Mack told me afterwards. If he had only told me earlier! Just recently I asked him why he hadn't told me he would wait for me. "You wouldn't have slept a wink," he teased, referring to my insomnia that has always plagued me.

I learned that Mack, too, had had a bout with insomnia during that time, his only encounter with the problem.

Mack and I are both God-loving, God-fearing individuals. Just as God had interceded to bring Ruth and Boaz together as well as Isaac and Rebekah, so I believe, He, through His providence, kept us for each other.

(When I read the above paragraph to my husband, he said, "I thought I was the only one who believed that.")

Neither of us considered my returning to college. We had had enough of separation. Instead of a B.S. degree, I would have an MRS. and "enter the University of Hard Knocks," Mack said. He thought he was kidding! Later, I earned more than the required number of credits for a college degree.

I immediately found myself in a predicament. I had another man's ring—not an engagement ring, but his class ring. I returned it immediately.

After that, I did a most stupid thing. One weekend, soon afterwards, when Mack was out of town, I went out on a double date. In all honesty I hardly knew how to avoid going, since we had been double-dating and I could not properly explain a refusal without divulging my secret.

I repented in sackcloth and ashes! I could hardly wait to confess to Mack. Not one word of reproof from him. Incredible! If he hadn't forgiven me, I would probably have committed suicide. Another man might have taken me home immediately—But this man was Mack.

That was my first discovery of Mack's complete discipline that characterizes his life.

Love and Marriage

"And the nights shall be filled with music and the cares
that infest the day shall fold their
tents like the Arabs and as silently steal away."
–Henry W. Longfellow

Mack and I were married January 18, 1941, at Glasgow, Kentucky. We stayed at an early tourist court called "Windmill Village." Each individual unit resembled a windmill. Romantic! I had seen the place the summer before and remarked, "That's where I want to honeymoon."

We traveled on to Nashville, Tennessee, for a few days. We returned to Monticello and to the only period of leisure in my life. We lived in Mack's bachelor quarters at the Cooper Hotel, operated by Jake and Nina Sandusky, for six idyllic weeks.

Thanks to the Dr. Tuttle's, we couldn't leave town to buy our furniture, since Mack was to deliver their expected baby. Patricia arrived one month after our marriage.

For our room and private bath plus three delicious meals a day (for two) we paid $40.00 a month!

Looking back, I wonder why we ever left that carefree place, but I'll admit I wanted the privacy of our own apartment.

As a bride, I had found myself the only female living among a dozen bachelors in that inn, one of them a former suitor.

Another roomer, an elderly gentleman, Mr. George Smith, I had known since childhood. He had ridden past our house daily on a fine horse on his way to check on a lease at Griffin. I had received many nickels from him.

After a trip to Louisville to purchase our furniture, we moved into the Hedrick Apartment House on the corner of Michigan Avenue and Vine Street, where we lived for three years.

Home

"Dear God, I ask Thee for no meaner pelf,
Than I not disappoint my self."
–H. D. Thoreau

Now that Mack and I had our own apartment, I could put my Home Economics skills, if any, into practice.

Because of my great desire to please my husband, I confess to a bit of anxiety in the kitchen. My fears had been unfounded. Mack likes all foods, "except pumpkin," and he even likes pumpkin chiffon pie.

I knew little of Wayne County until I started making calls with Mack. I learned he knew every road, creek, trail and hog path in the county.

When we came to a gate, I jumped out of the car, unlatched the gate, and rode the gate when it swung open—until one day a dilapidated gate fell flat with me. Thereafter, I inspected what I rode upon.

Yes, I accompanied him on night calls, except for cases of obstetrics, called "labor cases" by most patients.

The turning point of my night calls came one hot summer night. The doctor had been called some fifteen miles out in the county. I accompanied him. A passing motorist had fired into a group of pedestrians returning from church. One person had been killed. What a disquieting experience! After that, I became selective of calls.

We led a quiet, untroubled life—call it blind devotion or whatever—we were ecstatically happy. We each liked to quote from Edgar Allan Poe:

> *But our love it was stronger by far than the love*
> > *Of those who were older than we —*
> > *Of many far wiser than we —. . . ."*

Would I ever have to come down from Mt. Olympus?

The Doctor's Life

Dr. Roberts says:

When I graduated from medical school in 1932, I immediately became a country doctor and that nomenclature carried a large number of specialities. I became a family doctor, a surgeon, an obstetrician, a dermatologist, an otolaryngologist, an orthopedist, an ophthalmologist, etc. I also pulled teeth.

One day as I returned from a house call several miles out in the county, a family stopped me to see their 15-year-old son.

After getting the history and examining the lad, I told the parents I thought he had had pneumonia and had developed empyema (an accumulation of pus in the pleural cavity). I made this diagnosis by auscultation (use of a stethoscope) and percussion. We had no x-rays or antibiotics then.

I advised a thoracentesis—an operation which drains off the pus. This, of course, should be done in a hospital, but the nearest hospital was one hundred miles away.

The family asked me if I could do the operation at home. I told them it was no small task and asked them to take their son to a Lexington hospital. They insisted on my doing the surgery at the home. I had never done this procedure but had possibly seen it done.

I happened to have with me in my little black bag the necessary equipment for the undertaking.

After boiling my instrument, I asked the boy to turn on his side. I anesthetized with xylocaine a place in the posterior area of his lung between two ribs.

I made an incision with the scalpel, and introduced the trocar between the ribs and into the pleural cavity. Immediately a thick pus squirted all over everything.

I felt better already; I had made a correct diagnosis.

After the pus stopped draining, I inserted a rubber catheter through the trocar, then I pulled the trocar out, leaving the catheter in the pleural cavity. I put a clamp on it. I anchored the catheter with adhesive tape and put on a gauze dressing.

Daily, for two weeks, the patient came to my office. I would remove the clamp from the catheter and let the pus drain. I then irrigated the cavity with normal saline solution and applied a sterile dressing.

At the end of two weeks the pus stopped and the boy had begun to gain weight and regain his strength.

This might not have been the best procedure, but it was about all I could do. All I know is the boy lived, and I see him each Sunday morning at church.

[I (Alma) add: Following the influenza epidemic of 1922, my brother had double pneumonia and developed empyema. Our family doctor and my father accompanied my brother by train to Cincinnati for the same treatment.]

I had been called to Fall Creek in Wayne County on an obstetrical case. Everything went well, no problem with the delivery. The baby appeared normal—except that the contents of the abdomen, stomach, intestines and all, poured out into the bed.

The abdominal muscles had failed to close from the sternum to the bottom of the abdomen. I had never been in such a predicament!

I tried to get as much of the abdominal contents back into the cavity as possible. I then wrapped the area in gauze. I asked for a heavy bath towel. I rolled the infant in the towel and sent it to Dr. Morris Holtzclaw, a well-known surgeon, at the Somerset City Hospital in Somerset, Kentucky.

Dr. Holtzclaw did a wonderful repair on this anomaly. He and Dr. Robert McLeod, a pediatrician, took care of the infant until she was able to go home. They called her their "miracle baby."

I am deeply grateful to those two doctors for their skill and care.

A few years ago, I saw the "baby" again. She was grown, married, and had children of her own.

I had a patient, an elderly woman, who was not too cautious about what she said. Her husband was considerably younger than she, and his IQ similar to hers, probably not in the top 10%.

The couple had not been married very long until they began to have arguments and misunderstandings. One day the wife came into my office and said, "Doc, what would it cost to give my husband a kill or cure shot?"

"Well," I said, "I guess that would be worth about twenty dollars."

"I've only got ten dollars," she said. So that saved the man's life!

A woman came into my office a few years ago and said she wanted my advice on a matter. "I'll do whatever you say," she said.

I asked what the problem was.

"I have just found out my husband is courting another woman, and I want to know whether to sue him for a divorce or kill him."

I saved another man's life.

One day I had the misfortune to have two of my obstetrical patients to go into labor at the same time. The trouble was, they lived fifteen country miles apart.

I kept the road hot checking one, then the other patient. I feared they would deliver about the same time and I could not be present at both places simultaneously. I dared not tell either woman of my predicament for fear she would not let me leave.

The time wore on. I kept making my thirty-five to forty-minute trip, checking one patient then the other.

Well, it happened, as it usually did, the Lord was with me. One patient got ahead of the other one and delivered her baby in a routine manner.

I wasted no time in getting things in order and hurrying off to the waiting one. She, too, had a normal delivery. I was greatly thankful and relieved that everything turned out as it did. I later told the women of my plight.

Now that is not the end of the story. Three or four years later, the same two women delivered babies on the same day again.

World War II

Clouds lay on the horizon. Mack and I heard the ominous rumblings of another war in Europe. In the past, trouble in Europe usually meant trouble in our country.

Our World War I, fought to "end all wars," had ceased only a quarter of a century earlier.

In 1939, we had read with interest of Germany's conquests in Europe.

Now, allied with Germany and Italy, Japan virtually demanded the U.S. acceptance of Japanese supremacy in the Orient.

While we negotiated with the Japanese in Washington, D.C., they launched a sneak attack on our naval base at Pearl Harbor on December 7, 1941.

Germany and Italy supported Japan by declaring war on the United States, and we found ourselves fully plunged into the war—allied with Britain and Russia. France had already fallen to Hitler.

Our Draft Board went into overdrive. Older men beyond the draft age, joined by women, flocked to cities to work in defense plants or shipyards.

Monticello became a ghost town.

I remember when I passed through town one Saturday night (a night when everybody went to town), I saw only one male (no doubt a draft rejectee) on the street. I saw many females out that night.

Shortly after our involvement in the war, for the first time in history, enlistments were opened for women. The Women's Army Corps became known as the WAC.

Success of the early recruiting campaign inspired formation of women's organizations in other services: WAVES, SPARS, WASP and Marine Corps Reserve.

Because of gasoline rationing, all unnecessary travel came to a halt. As someone said, "We became a 10-mph town."

Physicians and farmers here in our county received "C" (unlimited) gas cards. The sick had to be cared for and food produced.

Though we lived on a main street, when we heard a car after bedtime, we knew it was someone for the doctor.

Food rationing included canned goods, sugar, seafood and imported goods, as well as soap. We learned to substitute honey and sorghum for sugar.

U-boats, those German submarines, sank boatload after boatload of bananas off the coast of Florida.

By this time Mack had become a <u>busy</u> doctor. He traveled far and near at all hours, even into adjacent Pulaski, McCreary and Clinton counties. The most dreaded trip, as far as I was concerned, was one across the Cumberland River, particularly at night. This was before the Wolf Creek Dam. That was a long trip over bad roads, and he had to be rowed across the river on a skiff by a patient's family.

Those were bittersweet years. Mack and I were together happily at last, but sad because of the daily war news.

Most every family was affected. My brother, who was just a kid, and my nephew were drafted. Mack had nephews in the army. Each service person's family lived in fear of having a Red Cross representative knock at its door with the news that a son or daughter had been "killed in action."

Kamikaze attacks terrorized the American fleet in the Pacific.

Just as all ears had turned to President Franklin D. Roosevelt by radio during the Depression, now we listened in rapt attention to him who had broken all precedent by being elected to a third term.

Our President reassured us. He emphasized that "all we have to fear is fear itself."

In England, the inimitable Prime Minister Winston Churchill warned the enemy:

> *We shall fight on the beaches . . .*
> *We shall fight in*
> *the fields and in the streets . . .*
> *We shall never surrender.*

We witnessed the day-by-day conflict through the eyes of our favorite war correspondent, Ernie Pyle. We were with him and "our boys" from the North African Campaign, Europe and the South Pacific until he himself made the supreme sacrifice near Bataan. We almost felt we had lost a member of the family.

Now We Are Three

On April 27, 1943, our first baby, Helen Dolen Roberts, was born at St. Joseph's Hospital in Lexington, Kentucky, where Mack had interned.

Only those who have had like experience understand our joy. What a precious addition to our family; now we were three.

"She's the prettiest baby in the nursery," Mack told me.

No longer did my husband receive all my attention and no one ever shared more willingly. Never had there been a more doting father.

The telephone woke Helen every time it rang in our one-bedroom apartment.

When our baby grew old enough to go out in a stroller, everyone heard us coming. Because of the war, rubber tires were unavailable; her stroller had wooden wheels that rattled on the sidewalks like a jolt wagon.

Helen kept me company when her father was out on calls. Many times when he delivered a baby, he was gone all day or all night or both.

I never knew in what difficulty Mack found himself. I stayed awake most nights until he returned. I prayed a lot.

We had our Victory Garden, and I did my share of preserving food. I enjoyed doing it; I was proud of my cellar. Freezers had not made their appearance. "Use it up, make it do, or do without" was a popular saying during the war. Americans readily complied with rationing measures, glad to be supportive of those fighting in the war. The courage at home was vital to the morale of our troops.

I pause here to say that perhaps nothing mirrors the mood of our times more than popular songs.

This, I think, has always been true. These melodies tell of the despair, confusion, struggles and hopes of millions.

Not only do they echo our thoughts, they depict an age or epoch, tell the American story: *Camp Town Races, A Bicycle Built for Two* etc.

They are furthermore used to taunt the enemy, defuse our gloom, steel us for conflict and sing of victory.

Perhaps no song has stirred more patriotism than George M. Cohan's *Over There*. A hit song in World War I, it again warned that "the Yanks are coming" in World War II.

Over There became the accepted phrase to describe the War, and the final sentence of the song, *"and we won't come back till it's over, over there"* had a ring of finality.

Other popular songs of the period were *There'll Be Bluebirds Over the White Cliffs of Dover, Praise the Lord and Pass the Ammunition, Don't Sit Under the Apple Tree (with anyone else but me), Deep in the Heart of Texas, Somebody Else is Taking My Place,* and *Blueberry Hill.*

On our 53rd Valentine Day together Mack gave me a Hummel Music Box that plays *"Don't Sit Under the Apple Tree with Anyone Else But Me!"* What a touching gift!

D-Day

"War is hell."
William Tecumseh Sherman

On the war continent, Hitler's army had proved invulnerable.

For months we knew a planned invasion of the continent by the Allies stationed in England was imminent. They prepared for the assault across the English Channel into Normandy. The questions were When? How? Where?

The code name of the operation was "Overlord." We knew it as "D-Day." "D-Day," what a foreboding expression! Did it mean death-day, destruction-day, doom-day—or please, God, deliverance-day? Time would tell. We, like the enemy, waited in dread and expectancy for that occurrence.

Every American old enough to remember anything remembers June 6, 1944. I remember it vividly. On that day we heard the radio announcement, "Early this morning units of the Allied Armies began landing on the coast of France." The die was cast.

We got our news through our open bathroom window from our neighbor's radio all the way across North Main Street. Because of gas rationing, traffic was minimal.

Fear was the universal emotion on D-Day. Yes, we turned to God in prayer.

We could not begin to visualize what was actually happening. The attack is considered by many as history's greatest invasion; never had there been a military operation on such a scale. What a day of bloodshed!

Our best strategy had been to delude our enemy by fictitious armies and the expected place of attack. A storm raged on the English Channel—hardly an ideal time to strike. We took a chance.

General Dwight D. Eisenhower used all means available. The Allies struck the enemy by land, sea and air simultaneously. By the end of D-Day 2,500 Allies were dead. Including the injured, total Allied casualties were almost 12,000.

Today, as I write this, we commemorate the 50th anniversary of D-Day, a tribute to those who served in that crusade to free the world from tyranny.

Now, we know the meaning of D-Day. It meant all the aforementioned; death, destruction and doom. But it also meant deliverance—deliverance from the Nazis' stranglehold in Europe. Thank you, God!

Eleven months later, Berlin fell.

A few years ago we visited the American Cemetery at Omaha Beach in Normandy and looked upon the thousands of marble crosses and Star of David monuments that stand in voiceless testimony to the cost of victory.

We walked among the graves reading dates on the headstones. The date June 6, 1944, recurred with terrible frequency; for most of those men, their first day of combat was their last. Interred there are 9,380 of the American soldiers killed in the Normandy invasion.

In no way can we calculate the grief, suffering and agony of those who survived. What a debt we owe, not only to those who fought in the Normandy Invasion, but to the men and women who participated so gallantly and sacrificially in the other campaigns: Iwo Jima, Midway, Saipan, Bataan, and North

Africa, Germany and all the other combat zones. Without the help of God, Great Britain, and the Soviets we would not have triumphed.

True to the words of the song, our service persons did not come home until it was "over, over there."

The war that Hitler instigated exceeded 15,000,000 killed and missing, including 292,100 Americans. The United States of America emerged the strongest, richest nation in the world.

Now We Are Four

"He blesses and blesses again."
–Alma Roberts

In 1944 we purchased a gray stone house on North Main Street. We lived there for thirty-six years.

I never dreamed we could be happier until on January 31, 1945, our second daughter, Ann Carol, arrived. Our happiness skyrocketed! Helen was twenty-one months old.

I must acknowledge after I had become a mother for the first time I felt if I ever had any more children I could not love them as much as I loved my first child.

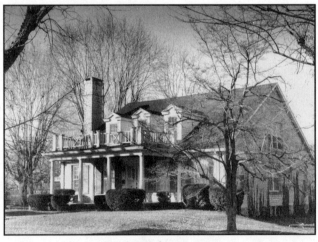

Our home for 36 years.

An old gardener clarified the problem for me. "Love," he said, "is like rhubarb; when it's divided, it multiplies." Exactly! Parents have hearts big enough to love individually and distinctively each child.

Mack recalls the night after Ann's birth. He was called to Chestnut Grove, near the Tennessee line.

"The night was frigid. I had crossed a creek. After I saw my patient and got into my car to return home, I discovered my front wheels were frozen. Instead of rolling they scooted. It took some time to thaw my wheels."

Milestones

In 1944 President Franklin Roosevelt had been elected to his 4th term. Suddenly, while the war was moving to a victorious close in Germany, the President was stricken by a cerebral hemorrhage and died almost immediately.

Vice President Harry S. Truman became president. The early months of his administration marked the end of the war in Europe. His decision to use the atomic bomb terminated the war in Japan and the Pacific on September 2, 1945.

The price of victory was too dear. Among those killed was Martin G. Shearer, my high school sweetheart. He was a fine, promising young man.

On a trip to London, I visited magnificent St. Paul's Cathedral. In one of the chapels of that great church I found Martin's name recorded among others who gave their lives in World War II for our freedom from fascism.

Now We Are Five

Our third baby, Marilyn Sue, arrived April 16, 1947. We had had three healthy babies in less than four years. Again, our cup of happiness overflowed.

"We had better start using single names for our children or we might run out of names," Mack said.

Perhaps the births of Ann and Marilyn contrasted with the usual picture during delivery. The expectant father did not pace the floor. In these two cases, the babies were delivered by a calm, expectant <u>father</u> in whom I had complete trust. That was the way I wanted it.

With three "babies" my busyness increased in geometrical progression. And Mack's?—he really began to hit his stride. He must have averaged working fifteen hours a day. Besides his office and homework he continued to make calls not only in Wayne County but in adjacent Pulaski, McCreary and Clinton counties.

As Norman Rockwell so well expressed it, *"We worked from fatigue to fatigue."*

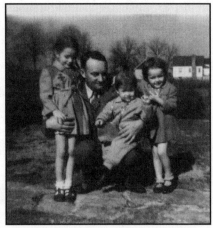

Now we are five, Robertses 1948.

Korean War

"I now know that wars don't end wars."
–Henry Ford

At the end of World War II in 1945 our GI's were returning home by the thousands. Following the hasty wartime marriages the next problem was a place to live. Prefabricated housing met this need. Then followed the "baby boom"!

Young couples fled to suburbia where many lived beyond their means, trying to "keep up with the Joneses."

The war produced a good byproduct in the G. I. Bill. It enabled veterans of World War II to attend college or technical school. About half of the veterans took advantage of the opportunity.

At the close of the war Eastern Europe was falling under the influence of the Soviet Union. The Soviet sphere became our adversary in every aspect of world affairs.

Soviet espionage was discovered in America. We discovered they had learned our atomic bomb secret and were soon producing nuclear weapons. Their aggression was too well known. The Cold War was on.

Now we had a new worry—the threat of nuclear war. Bomb shelters were provided and food stored.

Like a thunderbolt, the United States was again involved in war—in Korea. At the end of World War II, United States troops had occupied the Korean peninsula south of the 38th parallel, while the U.S.S.R. took over the north.

In June 1950, soldiers from North Korea stormed across the border forcing the South Koreans to retreat. The United States force came to their rescue.

We believed the Soviets had orchestrated the attack, and we moved to stop the aggressor.

General Douglas MacArthur who had been our chief military leader in the Pacific theater in World War II, devised a plan whereby Seoul was liberated, with the help of United Nations forces.

However, with the aid of Communist China, the war continued; no victory could be claimed.

General MacArthur proposed a solution with an all out war with China. President Truman fired the general, saying "I could no longer tolerate his all-out insubordination." President Truman feared we would eventually be drawn into a third world war.

Altogether, almost 1.5 million served in a war that continued for over three years. More than 54,000 of them died and twice that number were wounded. An estimated three million Koreans and Chinese were killed or wounded in a war that ravaged the country from end to end.

The Korean War was limited, unpopular and fought under the United Nations banner. In 1953 it was brought to an end without a clear victory.

Milestones

Back home the golden age of television triumphed. *Lucy* entered our living rooms along with Groucho Marx on the *You Bet Your Life* quiz show. We watched *Ozzie and Harriet*, *Dragnet*, starring Joe Webb as Friday, the *Ed Sullivan Show* and others.

In 1959, Alaska and Hawaii became our 49th and 50th states.

In 1960 John F. Kennedy was elected President of the United

States. He was assassinated three years later.

In 1965, Martin Luther King, Jr. led 3,000 protesters on the fifty-four mile march from Selma to Montgomery, Alabama, to muster support for a voting rights bill for blacks (The Voting Rights bill passed in 1965). In 1968 King was assassinated.

In 1968 Senator Robert Kennedy was assassinated.

In 1960 Harper Lee wrote *To Kill a Mockingbird*.

In 1969 we fulfilled President Kennedy's promise to land a man on the moon "before this decade is out."

When Neil Armstrong emerged from the space craft and touched the lunar surface, he said, "That's one small step for a man, one giant leap for mankind."

After having watched the moon landing, insomnia overtook me. I got out of bed that night in June, went outside and gazed at the moon in wonderment. Had we really placed men on the moon? Amazing!

The next day I related my experience to Mack. "Can you imagine the feelings of their wives?" I asked. "They stared at that moon, knowing their husbands were there." Mack said, "A lot of women would be glad to have their husbands on the moon."

Blood on the Porch, Dirty Diapers in the Driveway, Patients in My Hair

The Doctor's Duty

To cure occasionally
To relieve frequently
To comfort always.
–Anonymous

Dr. Roberts was never one to train his patients to keep office hours. Just as he made house calls at all hours, his patients called on him at all hours <u>at our home</u>.

When the doctor arrived home from the office in the afternoon, his patients awaited him in the driveway. Sometimes they had waited a long time, as discarded diapers testified. They continued to come—complaining of a sore throat, earache, bellyache, backache, and a leaping toothache. They had cold, "flu," and pneumonia. They came following accidents, wheezing with asthma and carrying a crying, croupy baby. You name it—they had the disease. Sometimes the patient had triple ailments. "Doc, I've got brownkitis, enkersema of the lungs, and dead nerves."

Callers came to ask the doctor to make house calls anywhere in the county or adjacent counties. We might as well have posted a sign: "Open 24 Hours" or "We Never Close."

Where else would you expect to find blood on the porch, bloody fingerprints around the knocker? How did the doctor feel about this?

He was very, very caring. He said that people could get sick or have accidents at any time. We had no hospital in our county during his first forty years of practice.

During those years many families out in the county had only one car or none. Patients had no way to get to the doctor's office until after the wage earner or farmer got home in the late afternoon.

How did the doctor's wife feel about these intrusions? I supported my husband. How did our daughters feel about it? They had never known anything else.

Mack and I empathized with patients in this situation—however, the privilege was often abused.

For me, whose idea of a home is a cottage small by a waterfall—without phone, television, doorbell or radio, I acknowledge this type of life required some adjustment.

I daresay no doctor has ever been more accessible to his patients. If there ever was a sense of calling to practice medicine, I think he heard it.

It's easy to remember the times in the summer when Mack had arrived home from work and had hoped to do some vegetable gardening. He would spend five minutes jerking and yanking the rope to start his garden tiller and about the time he got the tiller going, in drove a patient. Mack treated the patient and returned to his plowing only to have the interruption repeated time after time.

I felt sorry for Mack. Once, I tried to run the tiller for him. It had me all over the garden. "You're a little too light for the job," my husband quipped.

To say those callers were disruptive would be an understatement. Seldom did we have a meal when we didn't have to answer the phone or door. As our guests can attest, both host and hostess usually left the table—one answered the phone, the other answered the door. We would have expected such interruptions if we had entertained the president and the first lady. In later years, I set the phone on the table alongside the flatware at the doctor's place. That saved many steps. He also carried the phone in his hip pocket when he went to the garden.

I am not pitying us. Mack had chosen this lifestyle, and I had chosen him. He was wedded to his practice before he was wedded to me. (I was too enamored to do any bargaining!) We were young, energetic and ready for the challenge. Furthermore, it was our bread and butter.

Our patients became quite familiar. One summer evening as I washed dishes in the kitchen, I heard someone enter the front door. I knew Mack had a patient in the driveway, and I presumed it was he reentering the house.

Someone said, "I just thought I'd come in and see what you was doing." I looked around and saw a stranger—a farmer, a friendly, neighborly type.

We returned from a month's vacation to find a patient waiting in the driveway. How long had he waited?

We had a patient die from an asthma attack while on our porch. A baby was born in our driveway.

Patients who knew no telephone number but ours would call requesting me to call a taxi for them.

One patient often called on Sunday mornings asking the doctor to take her contribution to church.

A lonely widower whom I had never met, a patient of Mack's, sometimes called me just to chat, bless him.

Yes, the telephone callers described their symptoms to me when Mack was out. They often solicited advice. I didn't dispense much advice. One exception I recall. One Saturday afternoon a young woman called (the doctor was out) and said she was going to a drinking party that night. "I'm pregnant," she said. "Will it be all right for me to drink?"

I was equal to the occasion that time. Of course, I pointed out that drinking was dangerous to the fetus.

In 1960 Mack was having some angina. I urged him to slow down. Invariably when some caller came for him, he yielded to the persuasion and went out on a call.

"Let me answer the door," I insisted.

To the first caller I explained the situation. "Just tell Doc who it is," he said. "He never has turned me down."

Another caller who had received the same explanation said, "I've got the same thing; I don't pay any attention to it."

Patients came at all hours of the night. Mack saw strangers and all in our basement.

Believe me, our patients saw me at my worst, perspiration streaming down my face, wearing muddy shoes straight from the garden. One patient said, "I know one thing, you'll work." I considered that a compliment.

Dr. Roberts had always been attentive to his patients. They in turn have lavished him with gifts: quilts, afghans, cross-stitched and embroidered pillows, pillowcases and pictures, fruits and vegetables and birthday cakes. One dear lady cans green beans for us yearly. His patients have even included him in their wills.

I loved our patients—at least 98% of them. They became our best friends. That they had confidence in my husband was reward enough for me.

The Jeep

Nothing contributed as much to the rural practitioner's work as the four-wheel drive Jeep introduced during World War II.

Mack says "In our area, the problem in making home calls was not so much how fast you could go, but where you could go."

In an *American Magazine* article written in 1941, Gordon Gaskill breathlessly profiled the Jeep: "It can hurdle ditches, butt its way through the underbrush and run down inch-thick saplings as if they were hollyhocks. It can climb an angle that would scare a mountain goat; if it can't climb the outside wall of a skyscraper, it could probably make it via the stairway." I add my accolades. The Jeep all but gets down and claws and grunts.

Before the Jeep and WPA roads, a trip to Mt. Pisgah could be a day affair, sometimes reached by a detour through Tennessee. Now, one can drive to Mt. Pisgah easily in one-half hour.

How many miles Mack's Jeep—and he wore out several—saved him from walking, riding mule or horse, log wagon or other farm contraption, it would be hard to estimate.

I feared my husband was too daring, too trusting of the vehicle. Once when I traveled with him, after we had careened through mud holes, we went over a perpendicular hill that led to a farmhouse. I frantically exacted a promise from him that he would never travel that path again in a vehicle. Only the Lord kept us from going heels over head.

I will always be grateful for the Jeep.

Milestones—Desegregation

In 1951 President Truman integrated the military.

Due to the segregation in our schools and the resulting inequality for the blacks, an appeal was brought before the Supreme Court to desegregate the public schools. The 1955 court decision met with instant resistance. Championed by Senate Majority Leader Lyndon Johnson, a Civil Rights Act was passed in 1957. However, the struggle for civil rights was not over.

The first school to be integrated in the South was Griffin school—a school where Mack had formerly taught.

Teenagers let off steam in the 50's by their rock n' roll antics. Memphis' Elvis Presley brought rock n' roll its popularity much to the disgust of grandparents.

The movie industry, including stars such as Marilyn Monroe, Cary Grant, Audrey Hepburn, Gregory Peck and John Wayne, declined somewhat with television. However, drive-in theaters, frequented particularly by teenagers, revived the industry somewhat.

War-War-War

Vietnam

Our eighteen years of intervention in Vietnam culminated in our our most unpopular war—and one we did not win. The war was finally concluded during President Nixon's administration. It cost 150 billion dollars, and over 58,000 Americans paid the ultimate price.

The Gulf War

In 1990 Iraq's Saddam Hussein invaded Kuwait, thus imperiling our oil supplies. The United Nations General Assembly imposed sanctions. The United States organized Operation Desert Storm.

Operation Desert Storm began as an air war. High-tech bombs and missiles hit Iraqi targets. United States and United Nation forces routed enemy forces.

In the forty-two day air war and subsequent one hundred hour ground war, 148 Americans lost their lives. 100,000 Iraqi troops surrendered; some 100,000 Iraqis were killed. However, Saddam Hussein remained in power.

War on Babies (Abortion)

The war on innocent, unborn babies in the last twenty years has resulted in over thirty times more casualties than in <u>all</u> the wars we have fought as a nation.

Patience

How poor are those who have no patience;
what wound did ever heal but by degrees?
–William Shakespeare

Once, early in our marriage, when I perused Mack's thick medical books, I read, "A good obstetrician is one who has a big bottom and knows how to sit on it." In other words, a good obstetrician does not rush a delivery. "Patience will crack a rock."

Mack often carried a rifle in his car. Sometimes when on "labor cases," to pass the time while awaiting the baby's arrival, he did a little duck hunting.

I remember the first wild duck he brought in. He dressed it. I consulted my cookbook on the preparation.

The following day we had wild duck for lunch. Mack was out on a call, per usual. Helen and Ann were little tykes. They ate that duck with relish. I was almost afraid for them to eat that dark meat—looked like a "didapper" to me! I wouldn't taste it, and Mack missed out on the wild duck.

Such was the joy for the doctor, outdoor person that he was, of getting out of the office and into the countryside. He was always attuned to natural beauty. He has an eagle's eye, often calling my attention to things I have overlooked.

Nor did he ordinarily make a single house call out into remote areas. Just as he knew where everyone lived, so did the people in the region recognize "Doc's Jeep." On most occasions, neighbors waylaid him on his return trip and asked him to see an ailing person in the household. On numerous stops he treated not only one but two or three persons in the household. "Now Doc, will you check my blood pressure?"

Many, many times such calls were free. "People will usually pay, if they have the money," the doctor reasoned, "and if they don't have the money they can't pay." There were many notable exceptions.

This was all in a day's work and sometimes the "cares that infest the day" infested the nights as well.

A Typical Story

A former school superintendent tells the following story:

"I felt so bad I thought I was going to die. My wife called Dr. Roberts to our apartment that snowy night. Dr. Roberts sat down and visited awhile with us, no haste at all. He turned to me and said, 'You are not going to die.' He proceeded to check and treat me. By the time he left, I was practically well. I've told that story many times," he said.

Patients

Dr. Roberts speaks:

On a snowy winter day I traveled fifteen miles Mt. Pisgah to see a six-month-old baby.

The child had pneumonia and was running a temperature of 106 degrees axillary. The child was also having convulsions, probably due to the extremely high fever.

There was no hospital in our county at that time, but we did have antibiotics. I gave the patient a large dose of penicillin in the buttocks for infection, but we had to get that temperature down and get the seizures stopped.

I asked for a bath towel and a pan of ice water (which was no trouble to get). I wrung the towel out of the ice water and rolled the baby up in it.

I stayed around for thirty minutes or more and checked the temperature again. To my great delight and somewhat amazement, the thermometer registered 103 degrees. The temperature never went higher again. The seizures stopped. With the help of the penicillin and the Lord's goodness, the baby was soon well again.

Mr. Graham (not his name) had lived in our town only a few years. He was connected with a business firm. He came into my office and appeared quite depressed. He said he didn't know if I could help him. He had gone to several doctors but received no relief.

"What's the problem?" I asked.

"Doctor, this might be hard for you to understand, but I had a yellow tom cat that slept on my right arm for ten years. My cat died, and I was so torn up I was unable to sleep. That caused me to have a nervous breakdown. Can you help me?"

I empathized with my patient and advised him to get another tomcat.

I drove about fifteen miles out in the county, borrowed a horse and rode two miles up a mountain and delivered a baby.

"Doc," the father said, "I don't have no money to pay you, but I've got a couple of gallons of moonshine I've just fresh run off I'll give you." I refused the moonshine.

I delivered one of many children for a man in our neighborhood. He had no money. I had admired his guineas. He offered me a guinea in payment. When we tried to catch the guinea, it tried to fly over a picket fence and became impaled on one of the sharp stakes in the fence.

I lost that case by a guinea.

False alarms in the field of obstetrics were commonplace. I remember I was called to Denny Hollow one night to deliver a baby. They had had a recent rain. I attempted to cross the swollen creek and my car drowned out. A neighbor relative of the person who was having the baby was with me.

We were near the patient's house. The husband pulled us out of the water with his mules. The patient, however, was not in labor.

Patience and Impatience

As mentioned previously, some of our patients were the epitomes of patience. They would wait on the doctor for hours in our driveway, one parked behind another. I often had to ask them to move to allow me to get my car out to the street.

They also patiently awaited their turns in the reception room at the office, visiting and sharing symptoms as the cuckoo clock told the passing hours. Sometimes we had an extrovert who entertained, or crying kids who gave their mothers a rough time. Many patients read our magazines or the Bible, while keeping ears open to conversations.

Then there were the impatient ones. "Doctor should be in in five or ten minutes," I would tell a caller at our door. Away they zoomed in their car only to return five or ten minutes later.

I soon learned the older patients were the most impatient. I remember a ninety-three-year-old fellow who entered our overflowing waiting room. "You mean I have to wait on all these people?" he said. On the spur of the moment I gave an answer I have regretted: "Either you wait for them or they wait for you."

I ceased to be surprised when local women waiting in the office got up and went home before their turn in order not to miss their soap opera.

One morning Dr. Roberts was on a case of obstetrics at a nearby clinic. I had explained to the patients in the waiting room where he was and when he expected to return. One person didn't believe me so he popped up and walked all the way to the Monticello Clinic—only to learn the doctor was delivering a baby.

The same fellow upon arrival at the doctor's office would put his hand, missing three fingers, against the office window and peep in before entering the reception room.

The patients' <u>impatience</u> showed up again when people called the doctor to "Timbuktu." The doctor had scarcely left home before they called again—to see if he had started. I daresay that was impatience mixed with anxiety.

When patients came to our home at mealtime, the doctor left his meal to see them. When **I** answered the door, if the need were not urgent, I would tell them the doctor would see them <u>after</u> he finished eating. Dozens of times, those insistent callers would ring the doorbell again before the doctor completed his meal.

Some patients used him <u>only after office hours</u> or <u>only when they had no money</u>. "They're sick, too," the doctor said.

The Telephone

Someone has said your home may be your castle, but if you own a telephone your drawbridge is always out.

I recently talked to a friend who said he could call out on his phone but no one could call in. I have seen the time when I would have given half of what we owned for such a telephone and probably gone hungry.

I am inclined to agree with the person who wrote:

> *One telephone, necessity*
> *Two telephones, prosperity*
> *Three telephones, luxury*
> *Four telephones, affluence*
> *Five telephones, opulence*
> *No telephones, Paradise!*

Our telephone was off the hook twice—the first during Helen's home wedding and the second time when the girls were home from college for spring break and could not take the competition for their father on his afternoon off. They removed the receiver for a couple of hours.

In the Eye of the Storm

When you amble down any mountain path in Wayne County or visit any store in Monticello, you will probably find someone delivered by Dr. Mack Roberts.

During the breakneck years of the 1940s, 50s, 60s, 70s, and 80s, the doctor delivered more than 4,250 babies—90 percent of them home deliveries.

He delivered thirty-three babies in one December's mud, sleet and snow. He delivered three sets of twins in four days. He delivered four out of five sets of twins in one family—two sets within the same year. These childbirths were interspersed with his office work, home calls and tonsillectomies.

My role as dispatcher wasn't easy. Hundreds of times when the doctor returned from a call during the night I had another call for him—perhaps another case of obstetrics. Without touching bed, my spouse picked up both necessary bags and started again.

I would stand at the window and squint as his tail lights slowly disappeared into a fog as dense as a March snowstorm or listen to the clank of his chains on a snowy, rutted road. By that time my ever-present insomnia had triumphed. Sleep had left me just as surely as the doctor had gone.

When Mack delayed to return, the omnipresent worry surfaced. Is he up against a breech delivery? Is he bogged down in a muddy road or caught in a rising stream? Has he been held up? Did he drive over a bluff?

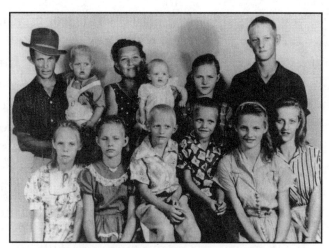

*Dr. Roberts delivered 4 out of 5 set of twins in the Preston
Bell Family—2 sets within the same year.*

Once, a friend who had seen the doctor pass called and said
he had been gone too long in a dangerous area. A neighbor and
I went in search of him. We met him coming home.

Another time my brother-in-law and I went to look for him
after he had been gone all day and night on a call. He had delivered a baby after a prolonged labor. I never learned to unknit
"the raveled sleeve of care."

Sometimes his delay in returning had been his choice. He
arrived home after breakfast one snowy morning in January,
having spent the night at Beaver Creek delivering a baby.
(Neither snow nor sleet could stop those little angels.) Later,
when I filled in the birth certificate, I noticed the baby had been
born at 2:30 a.m.

"That can't be right," I said. "You didn't get home until
after breakfast."

The doctor laughed. "It was such a bad night the family
begged me to go to bed and wait until daylight to go home," he
explained. Of course, they had fed him a big country breakfast.

I hear all sorts of tales from our friends. One lady said she was busy preparing breakfast—hot biscuits, country ham and such after the baby arrived at a friend's place. Dr. Roberts had said to her, "If you think I'm going home without breakfast, you are wrong." That was typical of him. He still talks about the "good fried turnips" he ate at Griffin fifty years ago.

Yes, we were often disappointed and had to cancel many plans due to our irregular hours. I never blamed my husband—a promise is a promise—first things first. PATIENTS.

I, of course, accompanied Mack on calls with prayer. I was not only the dispatcher, but many times I chauffeured him when our children were old enough to be left alone.

During one flu epidemic in March, I drove for him on house calls nightly from suppertime until midnight because he was exhausted. There was a reward—I got to be with my husband.

Perhaps no one better understood our home situation than our household helpers who came once or twice a week. Referring to the constant intrusive interruptions, one stopped the vacuum cleaner and said, "How you take this, I don't know."

Another said, "I told my husband I couldn't live with that—I'd leave."

With me there was no problem for the first fifty years of that rat race. I took it in my stride. We both were healthy and supremely happy.

Sure, there were days when I, as Eudora Welty said, would like to wake up and know that during the whole day the phone would not ring, the doorbell would not ring—even with good news—and that nobody would drop in.

That could wait until we retired. I, like Henry David Thoreau, had "several other lives to live." Hope springs eternal.

I remember the time when we were ready to go to the church for my mother's funeral. Mack got a call to deliver a baby. Dr. Robert Breeding came to our rescue and delivered the baby for the understanding (I hope) parents. I will forever be grateful to Dr. Breeding.

Two other tense times occurred when I was two weeks overdue. Mack was at Yamacraw, Ferguson, Brammer Ridge, Cartwright, Sand Cliff or Grape (across the Cumberland River) or elsewhere bringing a baby into the world for someone. But God, as usual, was with us.

Compressed into those busy years was the rearing and educating of our three daughters.

In His Office

The doctor has a secretary-receptionist, but he answers his own phone calls. He makes no appointments. Except for emergencies, he takes his patients in order as they come. Many times his waiting room overflows and patients wait on the porch or return later.

The doctor's office smells of antiseptic. Dr. Roberts wears a white coat. He has his own x-ray and fluoroscope. His bright spirit is contagious. Patients leave his office in a good mood. He jokes with them or farms with them. He knows them by name.

Some days he says he is "running a special" and charges them nothing or tells them to go to the Baptist Church, vote the Republican ticket and put their money in the Monticello Banking Company.

He might do a little art work on a patient, such as when he draws a cat on a child's leg with gentian violet after he has swabbed a cut, or acts as if he is going to sponge off the sleeve to give a shot.

He takes time to inflate a balloon for a child. He loves children; they love him. Their mothers have told me that they invent illness so they can "go see Dr. Roberts."

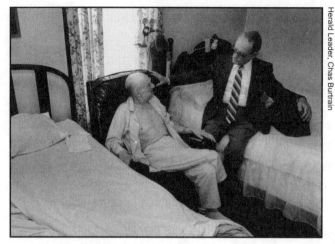

Herald Leader, Chas Burtrain

One of thousands of house calls.

It is impossible to describe his relationship with his patients. He couldn't pursue his work without dispensing his legendary wit. Nurse Jo Ann Crain said, "All the Valium in the world could not calm a patient like Dr. Roberts."

Always, on leaving, he tells the patients to let him know how they get along, and he means it. Many times he calls their homes to check on them.

Amusing Anecdotes

"Laugh and the world laughs with you . . . "
–Ella Wheeler Wilcox

Patients evoke all sorts of emotional responses from doctors. They sometimes amuse. For Mack no occurrence is so remote that he cannot recall it and relate it to every situation that occurs.

The Doctor speaks:
I was called to see a two-year-old patient in Newtown. The child was quite sick. About a half dozen women neighbors had gathered in to see about the child. Each offered her opinion as to what the trouble was. Their diagnosis ranged from worms to influenza.

The old grandfather amused me with his diagnosis: "I'll tell you what I think is wrong with the little <u>feller,</u>" he said. "I think he has had a nervous breakdown."

A man came into the office one day coughing and complaining of a summer cold. "Doc," he said, "I'd rather me and my wife both would have a cold in the winter than for me to <u>have one in the summer.</u>"

A man whose conversation was usually lubricated by lies had the answer for teaching a child to talk. Charles said that his baby had been bad sick, that the doctor had said he would never learn to talk. Charles said, "I knowed if he could learn to talk a tall he would be able to say cuss words. I set down on the floor with him and I had him saying d— in no time."

His Memory for Humor

Mack remembers:

My mother discovered that she and a visitor had a common acquaintance. My mother inquired of the fellow if he had had any recent news of their mutual friend.

The visitor spoke in a fine voice. "The last time we heard from her she was dead, but then we heard later that she was a little bit better."

A former neighbor was quite fond of his dog. The dog got sick and I asked about him. My neighbor said, "Her a little better. Her has got so her can knock about a little in the house."

When I was a child there was an epidemic of whooping cough in our neighborhood. Our father had all seven of his children immunized to prevent the dreaded disease.

We asked a neighbor who had several children if he was going to have his kids vaccinated.

"No!" he answered gruffly. "When I had the whooping cough, I had to cough and puke and I'll let them cough and puke."

A patient confided to me how he kept from taking a cold in the wintertime. He said he took no medication but he wore long underwear one week and the next week he wore short underwear. "Tharaway you'll never have a cold," he said.

After driving for twelve miles one night I rode a horse for three miles to reach a primipara who was in labor. I waited throughout the night.

The next morning about half a dozen neighboring women came in to help. Around noon my patient began to have hard labor pains, close together.

It was the custom for one woman to sit on one side of the foot of the bed and for another to sit on the opposite side. One held the patient's right hand, the other held her left hand and encouraged the patient to pull and strain down with every pain. (Doctors had straps that served the same purpose.)

Good progress was being made. The baby's head appeared, then wham! The bed collapsed!

Fortunately, with the help of the Lord, there now followed an uneventful birth!

Soon after I delivered a baby for a couple, the husband, Dick, came in for a prescription for his wife. He explained, "She is sick at her stomach, vomiting, can't keep any food down."

"Can she be pregnant?" I asked.

"Yeah, 'at the trouble. We did think we wouldn't have any more younguns for awhile, but we got to thinking they'd be a heap of company to one another. We decided we might have one every six months or so."

One hot summer night I was called to the Slickford community to deliver a baby. I arrived at the little mountain cabin up in the hollow some time before the baby arrived.

We discussed all the current events and caught up on the local happenings. To breach the silence, I asked the mother-to-be if she wanted a boy or a girl.

"I hope it is a d— wildcat and that it takes to the woods as soon as it is born," she said.

Parents brought a little boy into the office one morning—he had put a bean up his nose.

That evening the same parents appeared at our home with the twin brother. He had put a bean up his nose!

I drove about seven miles out in the county, crossed a swinging bridge and walked another mile to deliver a baby. The expectant parents lived in a two-room shack heated by a sheet-iron stove. The grandmother was present for the event.

After a short time a fine baby boy was born. It seemed to be customary to throw the father's hat into the fire when a son was born. So the grandmother grabbed the father's old dirty, oily hat and threw it into the stove.

The oil in the hat quickly ignited and suddenly there was a roar in the little stove. It became red hot, including the stove pipe, which was close to the ceiling. We had to close dampers to prevent a major disaster.

A neighbor called me to see her elderly mother, who had fallen. Upon examination, I found the old lady had broken her hip.

"I just told the Lord this morning if he had a cross for me to bear I was ready for it," the lady said.

"That is one time you should have been listening instead of talking," her quick-witted daughter said.

I have delivered two or three illegitimate children for a stark-naked mother. Every time she was in the nude—embarrassing even for a doctor, with neighboring women gathered in.

Jess, a faith-healer-type preacher, had a wife, Minnie, who had had a lot of sickness. Jess thought his wife complained too much.

"Trust up, just trust up," Jess continually admonished his wife.

One day Jess himself had rather severe pains in his abdomen. After he had agonized for a long time, Minnie said, "Jess, trust up and you will be all right."

"This pain is too low in my stomach for that," Jess said.

I had been to Newtown before office hours one morning to see a patient. On my way back to town, I picked up Jim, and gave him a ride to town.

"Somebody sick in Newtown?" he asked.

"Jack Tabor had a miscarriage," I said in jest.

"Pretty sick, is he? Think he'll get over it?"

"Yeah, I think he'll be all right if he takes care of himself."

Jim appeared to be in deep thought. We continued toward town.

"What did you say was wrong with him, Doc?"

"He had a miscarriage."

"He's been working up at that Hickory Mill lifting them heavy blocks—that's about what caused it," Jim said.

Shortly after Medicaid came into existence a patient came into my office suffering from "carditis" (continual use of free medical services regardless of need).

"What is your problem?" I asked.

"Doc, I've got bad kidney trouble."

"What are your symptoms?"

"Doc, when my water hits the ground it splatters and that's a bad sign, ain't it?"

"Yes, that's bad and that means you are in the final stages."

Slices of Life

I was called in the middle of the night to a small cabin half way up a mountain side to deliver a baby. This was one of the many times I wished I were elsewhere.

The delivery was normal—but the baby was far from the usual. The top part of the cranium had failed to develop. The baby had a face, nose, eyes and ears, but from there up was only the scalp with hair on it. In the medical profession, this is termed a "monster" or "frog." To my relief, the baby never breathed. I did not attempt to resuscitate it.

A year or so later, I delivered a normal baby to this mother. Then to my utter dismay, a couple of years later she had another "monster."

A small middle-aged man came into my office. He looked rather pale and depressed. He said he was sure he had cancer. "I want you to examine me, Doc, but I don't want you to tell my family about my cancer."

"How long have you had trouble and where is the cancer?" I asked.

"Three or four months, it's on my hip or buttock and it's getting bigger."

I had the patient to lie down on the examining table and pull his pants and underwear down. I soon saw what he was talking about. On his buttock was a dark mass about the size of the end of your finger. With gloved hand I took hold of the "mass," pulled it off and held it up for the patient to see.

"Here, Squire," I said, "is your cancer." It was a big dog tick. The patient was much pleased as well as surprised.

Several years ago a young man came into my office and asked if I would do him a favor. I asked what his problem was and he said he was married and had a family. The difficulty seemed to be that he had a girl friend on the side and she was pregnant. The fellow wanted me to give him something to get rid of (kill) the unborn baby.

I asked him to sit down and we would talk about it. I told him if I gave him something to destroy the unwanted child, I would be guilty of murder, he would be guilty of murder and the girl friend would be guilty of murder.

I pointed out to him that the act of abortion is worse than going out into the street and shooting a man, because the man might have a chance to fight back or escape. The innocent child could put up no resistance.

The fellow said, "I guess you're right. I guess that would be the unpardonable sin. I'd never thought about it like that."

I thought I'd done a good job. As the fellow went out the door, he turned and said, "Doc, I'll give you a hundred dollars if you'll do it."

The Doctor Speaks Concerning Abortion

"First, do no harm" - Hippocratic Oath

In medical school there were two fields of thought concerning abortion. If pregnancy became a threat to the mother's life, the Catholics believed in sacrificing the mother. The Protestant view was just the opposite. I'm happy to say I never had to make that decision. The issue of destroying the baby because it was unwanted was never considered. We in the medical profession were devoted to <u>saving life</u> rather than <u>destroying life</u>.

Strange Maladies

The patient who complained of a "diagram" headache.

Patient: "I'm sick at my stomach and have the scours."

Patient who had been to see a specialist: "He said I had cancer of the panther."

Patient: "Doc, I've got high blood pressure and rambling arthritis."

Patient: "Doc, I just terrify all night."

The patient who referred to his hemorrhoids as his "leroys."

Doctor in telephone conversation: "What seems to be wrong with him?"
Caller: "It must be something about his 'intentionals'."

More Humor

Doctor: "Where do you hurt?"
Patient: "Right here under the rafters."

The retired farmer was concerned about his "phosphated glands."

Menopausal woman: "I'm passing through the manifold."

Patient: "Doc, I've got distemper."
Doctor: "Horse or dog?"

Bystander: "They took Joe to Lexington to get a 'spacemaker'."

Doctor: "What have you been doing lately?"
Patient: "Nothing much. Been making a few antiques."

Doctor: "What seems to be your problem?"
Patient: "You're the doctor; you tell me."

A man wanted his tubes tied—"And I want it done before Christmas."

Patient: "I went to Lexington and they done a brain scam."

The doctor had performed a premarital blood test on a woman.
"Who are you marrying?" he asked.
Patient: "Leonard .... Oh, my Lord, I forgot his name."

Doctor: "Where is your pain?"
Patient: "My tail hurts."

Then there was the female patient who complained of "a weed
in my breast."

Elderly male patient: "Doc, they tell me I've got cancer of the
prostate, but it ain't spread to my ovaries yet."

Patient (leary of taking laxatives): "I don't want to get convicted
to anything."

Doctor: "How many children do you have?"
Father: "Dogged if I know, we got so many."

Doctor: "What does your husband do?"
Patient: "He don't work. He just 'draws'."

A woman came in to pay what she owed. After searching the
files, the doctor could not find a record of the debt. "What
was it for?" he asked.
Woman: "For delivering a baby."
Doctor: "How long has that been?"
Woman: "He's thirty-one years old."

Doctor: "What did your brother die from?"
Friend: "Cancer of the prosperous glands."

Doctor to wheezing woman: "You need greasing."

Patient in labor with first baby: "Dr. Roberts, I'm scared."
Doctor: "I'm scared, too."

Doctor: "Say you have an upset stomach? What did you have
    for supper?"
Patient: "Nothing unusual. All I had was nine sow's ears."

Three Bullets

One summer night around 1:30 a.m. someone knocked
loudly. The doctor answered the door. I heard the caller say he
had fallen out of a bunk bed down on Lake Cumberland and
had ripped his leg open. Mack sent him down the driveway to
our basement.

"Who is it?" I asked.

"I've never seen him before."

While the doctor dressed, I peered out the window. Three
Texas-sized men marched toward the basement. The doctor went
down to meet them.

A grown man fall out of bed? Was it a fabrication? About
that time our youngest teenage daughter, Marilyn, came out of
bed. The loud knock had awakened her. "What is it?" she asked.
I explained. She sensed my anxiety. Marilyn disappeared and
returned with a .22 rifle. "I have three cartridges," she said.

"How come three?" I asked.

"There are three of them, didn't you say?" Mack had taught
Marilyn to shoot a rifle that summer.

"I'm going to call the Police Department and tell them we
have three suspicious characters up here," I said. I called. We
waited.

About forty minutes later a police car cruised by. It turned just beyond our house in our neighbor's driveway and went back toward town without stopping.

The patient had lacerated his leg. The doctor worked on him over an hour.

My spouse was a bit surprised when he heard I had phoned the police. "How come, after all these years?"

"Because," I said, "times are getting worse. Besides, I always wondered what would happen if I called the police; now I know." I hasten to add that is not true of our present-day police department. They are quite vigilant. Commendable!

More Stories

Dr. Roberts remembers:

Seventy or eighty years ago when I was a lad, boys opted to go coon or 'possum hunting in the fall and early winter. This activity supplied much entertainment as well as a little cash if hunters were lucky enough to catch a few varmints.

Our neighbor, Tom, told us of being out hunting one night with his buddies. They heard Old Tige barking and knew he had treed. They all made a beeline to Tige.

On the way, the fellows began to try to figure out what kind of tree the dog had "treed up." One said, "I think it's a beech tree." Another said, "I believe it's a persimmon tree." A third reckoned it was a hickory tree.

Someone asked Noah what kind of tree he thought it was. "Well," Noah said, "the way he barks, sounds to me like Old Tige is barking up a stoopin' black oak."

One of my older colleagues, Dr. T. H. Gamblin, began medical practice in Wayne County around the turn of the 20th century. At that time we were infested with a bunch of "Quack Doctors" scattered about in rural areas.

Dr. Gamblin had been asked to see a patient who lived in a remote area, in consultation with another doctor, Dr. Zeke, we will call him. Dr. Gamblin supposed the fellow was a licensed doctor. He accepted the request.

Dr. Gamblin arrived at the patient's home at the specified time. While he waited for Dr. Zeke, who was an hour late, he went ahead and examined the patient.

A number of neighbors had gathered in for the occasion. Finally, someone announced, "The doctor is coming down the lane."

Dr. Zeke arrived in high top boots laced to the knees. He wore a long gray beard.

When the two doctors went out into the yard for their conference, most of the crowd clustered around them waiting to hear the diagnosis.

Dr. Zeke asked Dr. Gamblin what he thought the trouble was. Dr. Gamblin thought the patient had tuberculosis of the bowels. Dr. Zeke agreed and asked Dr. Gamblin how he proposed to treat the patient.

Dr. Gamblin outlined the method of treatment and asked what Dr. Zeke thought.

Dr. Zeke studied a few moments and then asked, "Have you ever tried a black cat skin poultice for such a case as this?"

Dr. Gamblin said he had to acknowledge he had never used one. "I saw right then that I had lost the respect of the crowd, so I packed up and left for Monticello."

Some few weeks later Dr. Gamblin met Dr. Zeke on the street and inquired about the patient. He learned the patient had died, but Dr. Zeke said, "I believe if I'd got there just a little bit sooner and got a poultice from a little blacker cat, I could have brought him out of it."

Back when blood tests were required for a marriage license, Bill, who worked in Indiana, came into my office one day to inquire about the law. He wondered if he could have his blood test made in Indiana, and if I could perform the blood test on his fiancée, Molly. They planned to be married in Wayne County.

Bill appeared anxious. I suspected he feared Molly might change her mind.

I told him I thought we could work things out. "When do you plan to marry?" I asked.

"She wants to put it off 'til Christmas, but I thought a good time would be 'long 'bout squirrel season."

In the early years of the 20th century we had some outstanding county fairs featuring, among other things, some excellent breeds of livestock.

Many times well-known farmers were appointed to judge certain rings of livestock. At one fair, three farmers were chosen to select the best bull.

Among the entries were a fine Angus bull, an outstanding Hereford bull and a top-quality Shorthorn bull.

There was also shown in the same ring a big lanky red and white pied bull with crooked horns 2 feet long.

The judges inspected the bulls carefully. They viewed them from different angles and discussed their good points. Two of the judges were in agreement.

"I'll tell you which bull I'd tie the blue ribbon on," the third man said, emphatically. He pointed at the lanky bull with the long horns. "That bull can whip any bull from Mt. Pisgah to the mouth of the Little South Fork."

Sketches

"What is your problem?" the doctor asked a patient.

"Doc, I'm hurting behind my eyes," He raised both fists and pointed his thumbs <u>toward his eyes,</u> "them two right thar."

We stop at a nursery to buy some plants. The doctor is hailed by a big guy, "Doc, you're the first person to see me naked."

The doorbell rings, "The doctor is on a call," I say.
"Can you write me a 'scription for a headache?" I prescribed aspirin.

A man came into the office with an empty pill bottle. "Them pills done me more good than anything I every taken," he said.
The prescription was for his wife's hormone tablets.

Patient—after the Pope had died: "I hope the next pope will be a Baptist."

Patient to doctor: "Heard you've been to Europe."
Doctor: "That's right."
Patient: "Did you drive through?"

Doctor to patient: "Say you are part Indian, how much?
Patient: "One-third."

Doctor to neighbor: "The less I charge, the less I lose."

Doctor: "Are you depressed?"
Patient: "Yeah. I was born in the Depression."

Doctor to neighbor lady who accompanied him to deliver a baby: "If I get a dime out of this, I'll give you half of it. She didn't get her nickel.

Then there was the patient who fed her cats on top of the bed.

Patient: "Doc, every time I took a dose of Dr. _____'s medicine,
    it blow me hat off."

The patient who called chloral hydrate capsules (green),
"lizard eggs."

There was one occasion when the doctor had delivered a
baby and the family was unable to <u>wake</u> the father to pay the
doctor.

Patient, speaking of twins: "I never saw two kids look so much
    alike in my life—especially Bob."

Patient: "Doc, do you remember that time you came up on our
    hill and I was frozen and you thawed me out?"
Doctor: "No."
Patient: "We had to walk a mile over our rocky road to the main
    road to catch the school bus. It was zero weather and I didn't
    have enough clothes on and I froze. I couldn't take a step.
    The school bus driver had my brother carry me home. They
    sent for you, Doc. You put me in a tub of warm water,
    wrapped me in blankets and everything and gradually
    thawed me out. Then I got pneumonia and almost died. You
    had to make four trips to see me."

The Optimist

The optimist fell ten stories, at each window bar
he shouted to his friends, "All right so far."
– Unknown

Dr. Mack Roberts is chief of optimists. He reminds me of the sun dial in France that reads, "I only mark the hours that shine." He evidently puts his mind in neutral, doubting nothing. He is like the fellow who had to cross a river before he could get a prescription filled. When asked how he would get across the stream he said, "I ain't there yet."

After Mack had surgery, I inquired daily about his progress. Every day he said he was better. After three weeks when I sensed his usual problem I asked, "How <u>much</u> better?"

"About two percent," he admitted.

My husband's irrepressible assurance contrasts greatly with my caution.

Recently, when we had started on a 250-mile trip, we had scarcely left the city limits when I heard a definite knock in the car coming from I knew not where.

Alarmed, I asked Mack if we shouldn't return home and have our car checked. "I can't hear it," he dismissed the problem.

A few miles later I complained the noise was worse. "It's getting farther apart," he said.

Farther down the road, I announced, "We're stopping in Albany to get this car checked."

"I think the noise will quit by then," the idealist claimed. Yes, there was trouble, but nothing major.

His ears ever attuned to the positive, he hears only what he wants to hear. He fills his conversation with wry cheerfulness and he practices the ancient injunction, "If you wish to live long, live slowly."

Happy person that he is, he is forever humming or singing. On his 89th birthday I heard him singing in the bathroom "Happy birthday to me."

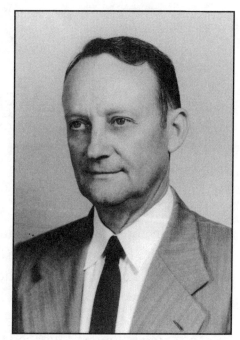

Dr. Mack Roberts

More Memories

Dr. Roberts speaks:

I was in the drugstore one day when a well-known alcoholic came in. He asked the price of skin bracer. When told the price, he said he would take all the drugstore had. Asked what he would do with so much skin bracer, he answered, "Shave my elephant."

The same fellow had webbed toes and fingers.

He was drafted for military service during World War I. When the doctor examined him, he remarked about his fingers and toes.

The draftee replied in a droll voice, "My great-grandmother was a goose."

One of my patients, whom I will call John, was a moonshiner in a remote section of the county.

John was called before Federal Judge Avery, I'll call him, in London, Kentucky. The judge had the name of being a strict no-nonsense judge.

When John was brought into the courtroom, Judge Avery asked, "Do you plead guilty or not guilty to this liquor-making charge?"

John answered, "I'm guilty, but you can't prove it on me."

The stern-faced judge said, "I don't have to prove it on you,

I'll just take your word for it." The judge let fall his gavel. "Two years in the penitentiary."

One of our Baptist preachers, a distant cousin of mine, was on his way to church one Sunday morning to fulfill his appointment.

He met a fellow whom he knew was on his way to get himself some whiskey.

After chatting awhile, the preacher said, "Well, I suppose you are on your way to get some of the devil's dishwater?"

"Yes, I guess so," the fellow said. "Do you want me to bring you back some moonshine?"

"Well, I don't know," the preacher said. "You might bring me back a couple of quarts of the dad-gummed stuff."

Some years ago, I made a house call south of Monticello to see an old gentleman, or you might call him "an old codger."

He was quite apprehensive about his physical condition. He thought he had a bad heart and that both legs were hollow and filled with water.

I examined him and found he had mild hypertension. I prescribed hypertension medication. I tried to assure him he wasn't in a serious condition and would soon be feeling better.

As I was leaving, he said, "Doc, I wouldn't care if you would take the old woman's blood pressure." This I did. Her blood pressure was considerably higher than his. I asked him if he wanted me to prescribe medicine for her, also.

"No, no. I've got her on a treatment," he said.

"What kind of treatment do you have her on?" I asked.

"Sassafact [sassafras] tea."

"Are you takin' any of it yourself?"

"No, no. I'm afraid to mess with it."

In World War I most of the moving of heavy equipment was done by mule power.

Mr. Bill Bradley, a native of Wayne County, tells of seeing a line of bogged-down mule teams in rain-soaked France.

Bradley said, "Along came a driver of four mules pulling a heavy load through mud knee deep. That driver surrounded and passed up everything. He drove on out to the main road and stopped."

Bradley complemented the teamster for his expertise.

"Hell fire," the driver said, "if you had pulled that Mill Sap Mountain as many times as I have, you could probably do it, too."

The driver was from Mt. Pisgah, just beyond Mill Sap Mountain in Wayne County.

One of my patients, a farmer who was about sixty years old, and his girlfriend decided to get married.

He had one of his neighbors drive him and his wife-to-be down to Byrdstown, Tennessee, to accomplish the event.

He wore a new pair of high-back overalls and had a big red bandanna in his hip pocket.

When they got to Byrdstown, they had to go on to Livingston, Tennessee, some twenty miles distance, to get a blood test. Then they returned to Byrdstown for the license.

Next they had to round up a preacher to perform the ceremony.

It was a hot July day, and the groom continually mopped perspiration off his face and neck using the handkerchief.

At last, a minister was found, and the vows were made.

All of this took a lot of time and a considerable amount of cash.

On the return trip, the groom remarked to his driver, "If I knowed it would take that long and cost that much, I would have just let it went."

Mr. Charlie Hedrick, a good friend and patient of mine who was also a prominent blacksmith in Monticello, told me this story.

He remembered one day around 1912 when there was a big 'political speaking' in town. J. W. C. Beckham, who later became governor of Kentucky, and Ollie James were the speech makers. The event took place one summer day at Doc Shearer's pond on Columbia Avenue, a place with plenty of shade and hitching room for the horses ridden by most attendants. There were few automobiles in the county at that time.

Many horses had lost shoes on the trip to town. Mr. Hedrick said he nailed on more shoes that day than in any day of his life—138 shoes. He received twenty cents for each shoe.

Uncle Will Phipps 1829-1918

Mack's Step-Great Grandfather

The Phipps family had migrated to Iowa. Will, the son, hoping to improve his financial condition, left his family in Kentucky for a season and joined his parents and siblings.

From the beginning, William did not find Iowa exactly to his liking, compared to his home state.

"The wind always blew," Will said. "If I took my hat off, it wasn't necessary to hang it on a nail on the porch wall. I could just place it against the wall, and it stayed there."

In 1882, the Grinnell Tornado struck. Houses were demolished, freight trains blown off the tracks, and trees stripped of their bark and branches and uprooted.

The storm killed Will's brother and injured several members of his family. Will himself was blown about fifteen rods and caught by a barbed wire fence. He received a thrashing by the wind. It beat him against the ground, bruised and wounded him. The wind tore his homespun "linsey woolen" clothing to shreds.

Will wrote his wife about the destruction. He promised, "If I ever get home, I'll never get farther away than Blevins' mill."

Neighbors made up money to buy the victim clothes. With the money, he bought a train ticket to Kentucky. When he boarded the train for the trip home, he turned and said to the wind, "Blow, blow, d____ you. You've taken your last blow at me."

On his trip he went into the dining car for breakfast. He was served poached eggs. He refused them. "I'm not used to sucking eggs," he told the waiter.

When William arrived in Kentucky and was asked about Iowa, he said, "I'd rather have one rock on the Little South Fork than the whole state of Iowa."

After his experience in the tornado, Will was terrified of storms. One day when a windstorm was brewing, Will's wife, Ursla, a domineering woman, ordered her frightened husband to go to the spring to get the milk and butter so they wouldn't be washed away.

William started, but when he got to the barn, he took a look at the cloud, and anticipated trouble. He was afraid to complete his mission.

He returned home. When Ursla inquired about the milk and butter, he said, "They're past Burnside by now." Burnside was a town several miles down the river.

Once Will had been summoned to serve on a jury for a murder case. When he returned home and told Ursla there had been a "hung" jury, she said, "Hung jury! I know what I'd 'a done to that culprit; I'd 'a hung him."

"Yes (expletives)," Uncle Will said, "but you'll never be called to serve on a jury; you always express your opinion."

Uncle Will was a great fiddler. He requested that his fiddle be buried with him. His wish was honored.

My Experiences

Loping backwards across the years, certain of Mack's patients stand out.

One, whom I shall call Bill, was an epileptic. He was a person of fine character—sometimes preached, though almost illiterate. He had a good memory. He often carried his Bible.

Bill became quite familiar. If we were away from home, Bill was often waiting for us—in the backyard—lying on the ground in the summertime or sitting on the basement steps.

He was among the scoffers who didn't believe man had been to the moon. Once when we were in Europe, Mack sent him a postcard. He wrote, "We are here on the moon and ready to shove off." Bill recited the message many times thereafter.

One of Bill's wives was short and fat. She looked pregnant. Bill had many doctors to see her—he believed she was pregnant. Once he called Mack, thinking she was in labor. It turned out she wasn't pregnant.

Later, Mack delivered a son for Bill's third wife. "What did he name it, 'Mack?'" I asked.

Yes, it was named for Mack and another friend.

I might say here that I was a bit dubious about the pay when Mack came in and said the new baby had been named for him. However, my fear was not always justified. Some boys were named for him because of the friendship between parents and doctor; Mack was honored.

One morning I opened the door of the reception room to call the next patient into the doctor's office.

"W. Jones," I called. A lad dropped out of his chair and walked <u>upright on his hands</u> into the inner office. But that's not all—from mid-abdomen down, the lower part of his torso was missing! I stared in disbelief. What a mystery that anyone could live in such a condition.

Years later I read about the courageous fellow. He was a student at Western Kentucky University.

Everyone is familiar with Leonardo da Vinci's portrait of a faintly smiling woman. What was the secret behind that mysterious smile?

Letta was the last patient in the reception room to be admitted to the doctor's office that afternoon. I filed charts as I waited for the doctor to be ready to go home. The woman, in her early forties I would presume, emerged from the doctor's office wearing that same enigmatic Mona Lisa smile.

When she left and I had closed the door behind her, I dashed into the office. "What did you tell her?" I demanded.

"I told her she is going to have a baby."

Now, I know Mona Lisa's secret.

Repartee

The doctor infuses his conversation with a touch of wit. He finds humor in commonplace happenings.

A few years ago, our librarian called around 11:00 a.m. and said that Mr. Gray, who had been a college boyfriend of mine, was at the county library. "He would like for you to come down to the library this afternoon and visit with him," the librarian said. (Mr. Gray's wife had died four weeks before.)

When Mack came in for lunch, I consulted him. "What would you do?"

Our daughter Helen had recently given me a bottle of Georgio perfume. Though Mack likes fragrances, Georgio was not among his favorites; in fact, he disliked it. Without a moment's hesitation, Mack said, "Put that Georgio on and go on down there."

On a European trip we spent the night in Rome along with our daughters. Helen, who had been in Italy previously, mentioned that one answered the phone in Italy by saying, "Pronto." Since our daughters, staying in another room, had the travel alarm, they were to wake us the next morning. We had gone to bed late. I had hardly gone to sleep when the telephone jingled. Mack reached for the phone, "Pronto," he answered.

In 1991 we made a trip out to Turkey Rock, a scenic overlook in southeastern Wayne County. We drove an hour through dense woods via Owl Town. Mack used to deliver many babies in that area and it is one trail I had never traveled.

After we had driven for some time, and I had kept my eyes open, I had seen no homes. I asked, "When do we know when we get to Owl Town?"

"When you see the courthouse," Mack said.

The hamlet that had flourished during the oil boom had vanished.

On our way to Florida for a vacation we stopped for a motel room in Marietta, Georgia.

"Yes, Suh," the affable innkeeper said, "I'll give you the room occupied by your governor, Governor Z. Grisham last week."

"Have you fumigated it?" the doctor teased.

The next year we stopped at the same motel. The same proprietor appeared. "Do you still have that room that was let to Governor Grisham last year?" Mack asked.

"Yes, Suh, and you are Dr. Roberts from Mt. Vernon, Kentucky (he almost got it right), and I remember what you said."

Tragedy

The Doctor speaks:

I had a family consisting of a bachelor and two spinsters who came to me frequently. They were regarded as respectable, law-abiding citizens.

They sold their farm and moved to town. I had heard talk that they were queer. They had been seen by a psychologist. I had never seen anything amiss in their behavior.

However, upon one occasion when they were in my office, one told me that a plane from Germany had landed in their back yard one night, bringing a doctor who had put a new heart in one of the women. This tale was corroborated by the other two adults. (This was before Dr. Barnard performed the first heart transplant.)

One night about 2:00 a.m. their neighbor called me to go to their home. When I arrived at the house blood was everywhere—on the bed, floor and wall. Evidently they had decided to end it all and the brother had been elected to perform the gory task.

One of the women lay dead from a slashed throat. Her sister was bleeding profusely from a lacerated throat; she was pale and weak. The brother, too, had a cut throat—but his wound was superficial. I finally got the bleeding stopped. I dressed their wounds and sent them to a hospital. The two had an uneventful recovery.

Home and Family

Some say the greatest legacy we can leave our children is happy memories. That is good. However, to me the greatest endowment besides love is to bring a child up in the nurture and admonition of the Lord and for parents to try to live godly before them, as the Bible ordains.

Bible training started early with our children. Always there were Bible stories, prayers, grace at mealtime and church attendance three times a week. We tried to instill in the children moral values and to teach them if we seek first the Kingdom of God and his righteousness, all necessary things will be provided by God.

We also taught them the work ethic—that no one owes them a living. We emphasized the need to be grateful and appreciative of help received and to show respect and compassion toward others.

We believed in discipline. "No" meant "No." Since their father was away so much, I became the main disciplinarian. I don't speak authoritatively, but at least we did a few things right.

Discipline is motivated by love. Love is the strongest force in the world. Our present-day idea of freedom of expression—all that matters is ME, is rapidly destroying our society.

Dr. Oliver Wendell Holmes was once asked when the training of the child began. "A hundred years before he is born," he said. "Begin with his grandparents."

Civility is a two-way street. Perhaps we get as much as we show. Teachers can profit in this field. I think good behavior is more likely to occur if our children know it is <u>expected</u> of them.

A loved child tries to live up to our expectations. Become involved in their lives, their projects. Never belittle a child. Set the proper example. Don't send your child to church—take your child to church.

Mack is a model father. No care was too menial for him—bathing, changing diapers, etc. Although the mother is supposed to know all the answers in infant care, Mack guided me. When Ann had the three-month colic and cried from 10:00 p.m. until 3:30 a.m., what would I have done without a doctor in the house?

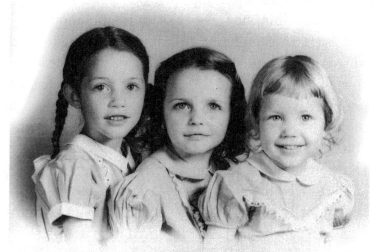

Our three girls (left to right) Helen, Ann, Marilyn

Mack played with the children, read to them, took them on calls with him, diapers and all, mainly to give me a reprieve.

Too, perhaps he was a bit indulgent. I remember well when we entered our youngest into grade school. When Mack transported her to school, she insisted that he enter the classroom with her. Then, she refused to stay at school. Three different times he brought her home, smiled and said, "Here is your girl." I had to return her to school.

Mack gloried in the academic achievements of our children and grandchildren. Instead of rewarding them for good grades, he awarded them when they made a bad grade. No wonder they are partial to him.

All three of our kids were in the school band. Their father attended their concerts as well as ball games, where they always played, when he could. It was a common occurrence for him to be called from a ball game by a policeman to make a call.

When the girls were in college, they received a note (usually written on a prescription pad) from their father about every time I wrote, which was often.

I found myself in the role of the traditional mother. First, a Christian, then a wife, mother, grandmother, caring for relatives and friends, as a cook, chauffeur, Sunday school teacher, and gardener. In the latter role, I had more than a suntan to show for my summer's work—two filled freezers plus shelves of canned goods.

I could have opted to teach school but decided to rear my children. Someone else might have done a better job, but none would have loved them as I did.

Rose Kennedy expressed my feelings, "I looked on child rearing not only as a work of love and duty but as a profession that was fully as interesting and challenging as any honorable profession in the world and one that demanded the best I could bring to it."

To me, "mothering" is like dying; you have to do it yourself. I am quite aware that I was fortunate to have the choice. Many, many mothers have no alternative but to work outside the home. However, it isn't always the <u>high cost</u> of living that motivates both parents to work, but many times the cost of <u>living high</u>.

We are all guilty! The deterioration of the home after mothers entered the work force, has played havoc with our society.

Our grandchildren, Tara Looney Swafford, Mark Looney, Aimee Looney Touchstone and Mack Drake, have added joy to our lives. Now we have two <u>great</u> grandsons, William Tyler Swafford and Thomas Alexander Swafford. God has blessed us repeatedly.

When our oldest grandchild, Tara, was brought for her first visit with us, Mack put a

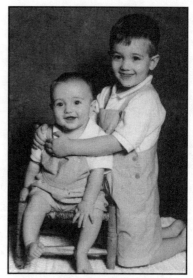

Thomas Swafford (age 1) and Tyler Swafford (age 3), great grandchildren

notice on our front door: "25¢ to peep. 50¢ to hold her."

Their grandfather set the grandchildren up with a special breed of cattle, polled Galloway. The grandkids continue to benefit by selling the offspring. When our youngest grandson, Mack Drake, arrived, our sweet Aimee gave him her first (unborn) calf for Christmas. Alas, the calf was born dead.

We made a special trip to Paris, Tennessee, to take Mark a peacock and two peahens from our farm at Mill Springs. Mark wanted to go into the peacock business. He lived in a suburb. What an adventure Mark had with his peafowls and neighbors! That prompted me to write a children's book about his adventures entitled "The Mirror Tree."

When Mack bathed Aimee, she said, "That's not the way Mamommy (her name for me) does it."

"Mamommy doesn't know everything," Mack said.

"Then why did you marry her?" Aimee asked.

Ponies

Ponies, one mare and a goat were the only pets we ever owned. Marilyn was "possessed" by the ponies–lived with them. I overheard her tell her sisters, "If you are ever frustrated just go to the pony lot." A Kentuckian, she has never outgrown her love for horses. She owns two mares presently.

Ann, too, was much attached to the ponies though she sustained all the injuries—a broken shoulder, a damaged knee that required surgery in later years while she was in pharmacy school. In spite of Ann's love for the ponies, she was my main helper in the kitchen.

Helen also was quite involved with the ponies—however, the majority of her time was spent reading or playing the piano.

The doting father bought five ponies for our children. The ponies multiplied. Mack was so possessed by his little girls he could not sell the foals.

"What about selling Caesar, Sputnik, Gentian Violet, and Pamper?" he would ask.

"No, no, Daddy. We can't sell them!"

"How about selling Piccolo Pete, Lazarus, Poison Ivy, Duke and Honeysuckle?"

"No, no, Daddy."

The ponies multiplied until we had fifty-three. We hired a person to care for them. Mack bought a double rig to drive the ponies in, and we had a trailer made to transport our finest ponies to county fairs.

The girls ran out of names for their ponies but their father did not; he came up with some doozies.

Mack bought a "pony" sight unseen after a smooth horse trader "buttered him up." "She's a fine white spotted pony," he had said. When delivered the <u>pony</u> looked like a work horse—not even a freckle on her. Mack promptly named her Hortense. My nephew, Roger, renamed her "Hornets."

We bred our mare, Bess, to Mighty Sun, a world champion walking horse. We had high expectations. The girls were away in college at the time. The filly arrived badly malformed. Her nose was misshaped and one hip out of alignment. We didn't have the heart to destroy her. I wondered what Mack would name our poor filly.

At that time, "My My" had won the Kentucky State Fair Championship in the five-gaited saddle ring for a number of consecutive years. Mack named our filly, "Oh My Goodness." We shortened the name to "Oh My." We gave her special attention and she lived four or five years.

Those were the good

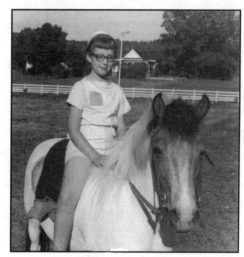

Marilyn on beloved Topper, first of 50+ ponies.

ole days, had there been no accidents. Later, Mack threatened to sell all fifty-three ponies and "throw in a pair of crutches." We finally, after the kids really grew up, sold a truck load of ponies, but kept the original ponies until they died.

Our Christmas Away from Home

Custom dictates that everyone comes home for Christmas. In our family not to have this period of love and celebration at home would be like celebrating the Armistice in Germany. What better investment can we leave our family than the ritual of tradition, whether plain or fancy?

It is mid-November, 1983. Already the atmosphere is super-charged with Christmas. We are off and running—but I, since my surgery a month earlier, only in the circuitous motion of my thoughts.

I have been in this predicament before, I tell myself. Previously, with faith and great expectations, I would shift into low gear and command myself, "To your tents, O Israel." Day by day I would call up enough strength to execute a page or two of my lists. But this year is different.

Mack sympathizes. "Christmas should come on February 29th," he says.

> To stop spinning my wheels, I stare out the window.
> Over the woodlands brown and bare
> Over the harvest fields forsaken
> Silent, and soft, and slow
> Descends the snow.
>
> *Longfellow*

The doorbell rings. My gardener hands me pine cones for my basket on the hearth. "I thought you might like some holly and pine branches, too," he says. His eyes twinkle and his gnarled hands are ungloved. He knows his gift is forthcoming— but he is an amiable fellow.

The fragrance of the evergreens triggers treasured memories of past Yules, as when our oldest daughter, Helen, scorned the mention of an artificial tree and quoted Robert Frost.

> But tree by charity is not the same
> As tree by enterprise and expedition.

We would go off across streams and Christmas scented forests to search out the perfect tree. I recall the year Grandfather, ax on shoulder, stumbled with us over hillsides and the girls would call, "Up here, look at this one, Grandpa; down here, Grandpa, I've found one"; or the year when we placed the tree in the playpen. (The baby wouldn't stay in it.)

As the twilight turns into darkness, I'm in the Valley of Doubts. Can I?

The telephone arouses me, "Mama," Ann says, "I'm calling to tell you we're celebrating Christmas at my house this year. You looked rested the last time I saw you; but if you go through Christmas you won't." I protest: "You don't have the time, the grandchildren will be disappointed and I can manage. I am feeling stronger."

Ann was as persistent as Br'er Rabbit striking the Tar Baby. "I have three teenagers to help me. Please, Mama, Daddy will be on my side, won't you, Daddy?" Mack is all for it, and it is not February 29th.

I try to sleep on it. I wake early. Over a cup of tea, I watch, through the window, a tufted titmouse. He comes fearlessly to the sunflower feeder, nips up a seed, takes it to the deck railing, whacks it open, then flits to the suet cone, sampling and chirping happily. Could I sample, too? Accept the invitation, enjoy, enjoy.

The thought vanishes as quickly as the tomtit.

In our household no one likes change. I reason: Setting traditions adds a new dimension to our lives. Nothing is much worse than skimpy traditions. Besides, Mack and I need that annual excitement in our lives. What are grandparents for! It's not the length but quality of life that counts. Responsibility had a hold on me like Scotch tape on wrapping paper. And always in my subconscious mind I wonder if there will be a change, an illness or death another year.

To alleviate my turmoil I rationalize that anticipation of the labor is usually worse than the real thing. I am used to running on adrenalin. I will have a kitchenful of daughters cleaning up after I have prepared the food. And, I add, with the grandchildren running hither and yon.

No, I am not immune to the Christmas spirit. To me Yuletide is a sentimental trip. Christmas lights, snowy nights, city streets, happy crowds. Dickens expressed my feelings. "There is no other time of the year when excitement is more heady, emotions more powerful, secrecy more condoned, love more in evidence." In my Journal each Christmas has been recorded, "Another joyful, blessed Christmas."

The entire family try to persuade me to accept Ann's invitation. Then, the right side of my brain, or is it the left? says, "Just think, without all that work what you could do. Shouldn't I, when the body says 'slow down', listen to it?" Then, the other side of my brain questions, "Would a Tennessee Christmas measure up to a Kentucky Christmas?" I'm a White Christmas person. Little chance for a White Christmas in Tennessee.

I debate the proposition.

Again, I'm supersaturated with painful indecision. Of

course, the new plan won't eliminate the gift buying. However, most of that is behind me. I am an early shopper, and I am able to gift wrap.

I am greatly tempted to capitulate when it occurs to me that I can escape decorating. Oh, Doo-Dah, day! I must not be all woman when it comes to that. I detest it, but there are those all-important memories at stake again. I would miss planning innovative entertainment for the occasion. One year we instituted a Cobweb Party in which colored yarn fastened to gifts was strung across the room, attached to high poster beds or armoires and such until it indeed did present a colorful cobweb. What fun to crawl and straddle through the network of string, rolling the strands as we progressed to the hidden gift! The children liked it so much it has become a yearly ritual. Another Christmas we smashed a pinata. Toys and candy flew all over the basement to the delight of the kids. At a different time we had Christmas crackers, straight from England—those gaily wrapped "firecrackers" containing fortunes. Last year, the grandchildren sipped mocktails of my own grapejuice from whistling sake cups. I always hoped that these things would be a sort of souvenirs of the past for our offspring.

Mack senses my anxiety. He reads to me from a magazine. "No one ever choked to death from swallowing her pride. Try coasting this year," he suggests.

"The good life is active, not passive," I reply.

Yet, it would be a culmination of a dream come true, to have the liberty, the independence and the flexibility of stepping to the tune of my own drummer this joyful season.

"I have three helpers, Mama," echoes in my thoughts.

The third phone call convinces me when Ann says, "Just this year."

With a sudden sense of freedom that was liberating yet guilt laden, my mind whirled counterclockwise. I would learn the pleasures of Christmas. It is the Year of the Jubilee, take advantage, be glad!

Immediately, I plan a little get-together for neglected friends. Now I would watch Christmas specials on television. I would attend programs that I had formerly not even hoped to enjoy.

For a change, I reveled in shopping, without haste, and delighted in the spirit of the excitement, hustle and bustle of the magical season. I slowed down and appreciated the artful displays. I stepped to the rhythm of blaring Christmas music rather than getting ahead of the beat. I visited the nursing home, taking little gifts to known patients. It was beginning to feel a lot like Christmas.

A stimulating afterthought: If I were going to celebrate this year, I would do it right. No special holiday cleaning, no brass or silver polishing, no digging in the closets for decorations— no tree. I'd let both body and soul idle. Just label me "Scrooge."

The time arrives for our five-hour trip. Mack loads our Oldsmobile to capacity with gifts, and there also travel with us a baked country ham, loaves of homemade bread, beet pickles, grape juice, jam cake and a Christmas trifle.

Sadly, we leave our home ticking with memories! There was that basket of pine cones on the hearth.

The sky is overcast.

We pass houses with Christmas lights blinking; some are outlined in multicolored lights. Those people must be the opposite of Scrooge or own the light company.

In a short time rain sets in. Horses stand like statues, outside open barn doors, taking the cold rain. Cattle huddle with backs to the wind. Half-drowned chickens dash for shelter. The rain beats harder, making driving difficult. We use our headlights. It's a wet-feet day.

"What if we had a flat?" Mack jolts me to life. "How would we ever get to the spare underneath the gifts in this drenching downpour?"

I try to change the subject. I flip on the radio. *"There's no place like home for the holidays,"* assails my ears. I turn to another station.

Now the countryside is wearing ponds in lowlands.

Our wiper blades are not performing well. "Some areas in Memphis are already flooded," the station announcer informs us.

At last, we pull into our daughter's circular driveway in Paris, Tennessee. The colonial style house is ablaze with lights. The windows display handmade wreaths.

We are the last arrivals. Grandchildren, daughters and sons-in-law hail us with "Merry Christmas!" The phrase has a new meaning, now.

We are not allowed to help unload.

There is no stamping of snow, rather the shedding of raincoats and umbrellas. Instead of swirling snow, there is swirling rain.

The house is alive with excitement. In the foyer a pine tree, fresh from the forest, brushes the ceiling. I had years ago succumbed to the phony ones. It is laden with Ann's hand-wrought ornaments.

The home is dressed in hollies, ivy and mistletoe; nothing has been omitted. Someone has spent days decorating—I know, Aimee—she's the artistic granddaughter. (For a second, reality returns in my thoughts. I'd hate to have to dismantle everything.)

Christmas aromas emanate from the kitchen.

In front of a crackling fire they ply us with hot, spiced tea. It is just the beginning of the cosseting we receive. Brass and copper shine in the dancing firelight. The rain is forgotten in the comfort of the cheer. Now, my conscience only whispers.

My efforts to help are firmly rejected. I am a guest! I see copies of my treasured holiday recipes on the kitchen counter. (Is my kitchen enjoying its sabbatical?)

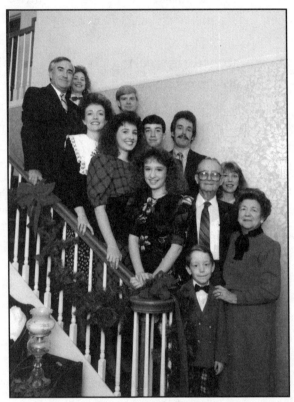

Family togetherness at Christmas time
Christmas at the Looney's 1987.

Strangely enough I do not have total recall of the evening and following day. But each in turn progressed as smoothly as a brook flowing over pebbles.

And that banquet, the one to make mine forgotten, appeared effortless on my part and praiseworthy on the part of Ann and her children. It was garnished by the cheer of conversation.

I remember the impeccable table, with the Belgian cut-work tablecloth (I no longer used mine-who would iron it?); the gentlest flickers of candlelight from crystal candelabras; the Christmas touches, not overdone, even to the small individual gingerbread houses that served as place cards! All were made by our artsy-craftsy Aimee. They would be placed in the freezer and used again. Would we be the pampered guests?

What a hostess! Was she trying to outdo me? Why had I worried? Tradition was followed, even to the Cobweb Party. And I didn't have to clean up the mess.

At last a brief winter day had ended. In our assigned bedroom, Mack peers out the window, "Is it white?" I ask. "100% cats and dogs," he answers. The rain had not been heard for the bustle of the household. Tranquility settles warm over us like an electric blanket and we dream of wet Christmases.

On our trip home the second day, in our blissful aloneness, I reflect that despite myself, my experience has exceeded my expectations. Ann's celebration was exactly the type of festivity I had aspired for and never attained.

A tranquil silence settles between Mack and me, but loneliness sets in. There is nothing quite so empty as that after-Christmas feeling, and I can almost feel the year slipping away.

We travel a polished world. It continues to rain intermittently, but wet Christmases, we have learned, can have a charm of their own.

I glance at my hands and behold my nail polish intact!

I find myself telling Mack that there are some things in life we just have to adjust to and not try to arrange everything to our own specifications.

He smiles.

Togetherness

Mack may have made, to use a phrase from Dizzy Dean, the "wrong mistake" when he married me, but our marriage was for keeps. Love is the mortar that holds two people together.

I realize the world is not full of people of Mack's stature and I consider it a special honor to have loved and shared his life for fifty-nine years.

"Let there be spaces in your togetherness," Kahil Gibran advises in keeping marriage harmonious—no problem there.

Someone has said that we cannot really love anybody at whom we never laugh.

Mack's busyness never checked the flow of his cheerful spirit. He announces his presence by singing or whistling.

When we built our new home in 1979, I handled the paper-work. At the end of the first month of our project, I said that I needed a secretary. "What you need," Mack said, "is a treasurer, and let me pick her out."

My spouse has given me everything gift-wise including a new Cadillac "for having the shingles." He gave me freedom and support to listen to my drummer, no matter what my age. But his gift of <u>self</u> was best. He ensures my happiness by just being there.

"You make my world go round," I told him.

"Clockwise or counterclockwise?"

I am in love with the comfort of our home. Home offers the

peace I find nowhere else. It is my escape hatch. I always thought a criterion of a good marriage was contentment at home with one's beloved; I still think that.

We are not too old or lazy for candlelight dinners for two at home (it might be high noon on a dreary day) or for picnics out in the backwoods we know well.

However, to keep our sanity, there were times when we had to get away—to come up for air. Mack recently mentioned having seen twenty-three patients who came to our home one Sunday morning before church time; that triggered a vacation.

Usually within ten minutes after we returned from a trip, we were jolted back to reality. I sometimes repented of having returned at all. Again, the "Philistines were upon us." (I'm only kidding.) I, who liked to have a wide margin in my life, found I had no margin at all.

Aristotle Onassis, one of the world's wealthiest men, said, "The greatest luxury in life is privacy." He knew more than just how to make money.

I received many bouquets from my husband—not from the florist, but rare bouquets of such wild flowers as the mountain laurel (the natives call it "ivy"), flame azaleas, called also wild honeysuckle, and rhododendron.

To get those flowers, Mack left the Jeep parked on the ridge road at Brammer Ridge or some other place out in the county. He clung to trees and bushes, slipped and stumbled as he descended the rocky slope at the risk of a fall. Flowers obtained, he pulled, yanked and grasped whatever lent support, to climb back to the roadway with his flowers.

Those pink and white faceted clusters of the laurel, "born to blush unseen and waste its sweetness on the desert air," placed in a vase, delighted us for a week. A little harvesting did them no harm. Mack's thoughtfulness was greatly appreciated.

Travel

In February 1948, Mack came in late for lunch, per usual. He said, "Get the young'uns ready, we're going to take a vacation."

A vacation? We had never had a vacation, and time off from work had never entered our minds—at least not <u>Mack's</u> mind. "Whatever happened?" I asked.

My spouse had read an article in a medical journal, "H Stands for Heart Disease." The article told of a driven physician who had never once taken time off for a vacation. "Last week his will was probated," the article said. The doctor had died from a heart attack.

"Where would we go?" I wasn't averse to the idea.

"Where but Florida? Dr. Rankin says 'If a man had as much sense as a wild goose he would go south in the winter'," my husband said and smiled.

We had been having typical Febru-r-rary weather. The doctor had been working day and night. I found it mind-boggling to think of getting three children ages ten months, three and minus four years ready for a twelve-day trip. How could I take enough clean clothes? There were no Laundromats. Diapers? Yes, I had seen Chux disposable diapers at the drugstore. I supposed they would serve the purpose, though we used soft birdseye or gauze diapers. Twice I had had two babies in diapers at the same time. I could fold diapers in my sleep.

As I went about making lists, getting warm-weather clothes

ready, rounding up picture books, crayons and readying the house, it occurred to me it would be easier to bring Florida to us. Neither Mack nor I had been south of Nashville.

Finally, all packed, we leave home around ten o'clock. one February morning—not exactly a jump start.

We leave Kentucky farmers burning tobacco beds, getting ready for another cash crop. We run into snow before we reach Oneida, Tennessee, and have to have our tire chains put on our new blue and white Chevrolet.

We eat our packed lunch at Oakdale, Tennessee, then travel southeast, chains rattling, on Highway 27 toward Chattanooga. A distance down the road we run out of snow and are able to shed our tire chains.

Now we pass through Tennessee valleys and piney woods noting "See Rock City" signs on barns. We drive through Harriman, Spring City, Dayton, Soddy and Daisy and arrive at Chattanooga with its Lookout Mountain. The children are quite taken with the Chattanooga Tunnel.

After entering Georgia, we follow our Triple A routing toward Dalton, Georgia. We make our acquaintance with carpet factories and textile mills. Chenille bedspreads seem to line the roadsides in northern Georgia.

We begin to notice the red clay banks of Georgia. Our narrow road takes us through the center of every sleepy town on our route, characterized by large white frame houses off the ground (for ventilation?). Each town has its own antebellum homes with distinctive white columned verandas. Signs invite us to see Stone Mountain and Beautiful Calloway Gardens.

We arrive at Atlanta after dark and get a motel room in the south side of town. We discover we have a sick baby. The sick child turns into a very sick child. Thank goodness there was a doctor in the house.

On the road again the next morning, our second night's destination is Jacksonville, Florida (we didn't realize Georgia was such a big state!). We drive about 40 mph—little traffic, few trucks and no interstates.

We are greatly impressed with the pecan groves with black Angus cattle feeding on the green grass.

We crisscross the area devastated by Sherman's famous "march to the sea."

Now and then, passing through a wooded area, we glimpse a cart pulled by two lumbering mules hauling in resin from tapped pine trees.

Another not so pleasant sight is the road maintenance crew—prisoners, some in shackles, overseen by a boss with a shotgun on his shoulder. Those men didn't stand and lean on their shovels. Believe me, they worked!

Stuckey's Pecan Shoppes with their "clean restroom" signs beckon us. We learned it paid to stop every 100 miles to feed and exercise the kids.

We continue southward. Davis Brothers Motels invite us to spend the night with them, but we are bound for Jacksonville.

Our children are tired, irritable, "When do we get there? She touched me. I have to go to the bathroom." They scramble back and forth from front seat to back seat (no seat belts). (If we had only had a minivan!)

The day turns into night. We are still fighting the battle of Georgia. What a big state!

We are worried about our toddler. We give her medicine faithfully.

I hear our three-year-old, Ann, ask her sister, "Hella, do you like Georgus?" It was dark as it would get. "No," Helen says. I agreed.

At last, Jacksonville lights are visible. Five tired travelers, one very sick, turn in for the night at an inn. The third day finds our sick one no better.

Northern Florida welcomes us with greenness. We come across cypress swamps. We see a stork standing on one leg. "Look, children, look." Palmettos and live oaks draped with Spanish moss are new to us.

We travel on highway A1A, the coastal highway, and arrive at charming historical St. Augustine. We drink from the Fountain of Youth and get our first glimpse of the Atlantic Ocean.

Ditches on either side of the road are filled with dark water. Occasionally we see someone sitting on the bank dangling a line in the water. Razor-backed hogs and skinny cattle roam the roadside. There are no stock laws.

Heading south, near Ocala, we meet spring. Blooming dogwoods welcome us. Under a turquoise sky, the weather is warmer. We roll down our car windows. We have no air conditioning.

Pastel motels with tiled roofs and jalousies line the roadside. They wear such names as The Flamingo, The Sandpiper, The Driftwood, and Sage and Sand. They usually have a sparkling pool, waving palms, umbrella tables with aluminum lawn chairs with colorful webbing, and shuffleboard courts. Wind chimes tinkle noisily.

The worst signs we encounter on our trip are the "no vacancy" signs. We have no reservations. For an overnight stay at a motel we usually paid seven or eight dollars.

Now we are in the lake and orange country. Beautiful! We are surprised to see ripe oranges on the same trees bearing fragrant orange blossoms.

We have hit the weather just right. We have come from snow to summertime. Our two-lane road is a black, blistering ribbon. Look out for sunburns!

We stop at a fruit stand that advertises orange juice. "All U can drink for 10¢." We do the sign justice and buy some sweet tree-ripened fruit to take with us. The kids don't want to get back into the car.

"Sunshine and orange juice," the doctor seemed to think was a magical combination. He didn't mention the <u>sand</u> in our shoes.

We pass through miles and miles of barren, uninhabited, monotonous countryside. Now and then we see a half starved humpbacked cow wandering aimlessly.

The girls whine.

"Color in your coloring books," I suggest, but the crayons have melted in the window.

"Mama, she threw a book out the window."

We back up to pick up the picture book.

Though we have hoped to stay at Hollywood, Florida, because our baby is so sick we stop early and stay at the red-tile roof Spanish Courts in Riviera Beach just north of West Palm Beach. Would we have to hospitalize our baby?

In a day or so our sick one has improved greatly and we travel on to Miami. We find no accommodation—except a motel room on the Tamiami Trail for $22 a night. That is too high for us. We return to West Palm Beach and found a room.

Now we have another sick child—a homesick child. "I want to go home where Suzanne [her doll] is," Ann says, "and play Santas Claus is coming to town."

Next day we visit elegant Palm Beach. We shop on ritzy Worth Avenue and see Empress Josephine's tiara in a jewelry store window!

We pass by the fabulous Breakers Hotel where one of the Rockfellers is honeymooning. We see a man transporting a "lady" in a jinrikisha.

While dining in restaurants, we discover that we are the <u>youngest</u> vacationers.

We visit the beach for the first time and build sand castles. "Where is your pail?" I ask Ann. "A wave swallowed it!"

Back in Central Florida we take a glass-bottom boat ride at Silver Springs and visit Cyprus Gardens as well as Bok Tower. We enjoy a carriage ride to the Alligator Farm at Jacksonville.

Returning through Georgia, we are fortunate to see the peach orchards in bloom.

We are happy to reach Kentucky and especially home. We have traveled more than 2,000 miles and have spent thirty -nine dollars for gas.

They say a change is as good as a rest. We had had a great change. That first trip had been traumatic.

Later vacations were as Dr. Samuel Johnson said about second marriages—the triumph of hope over experience.

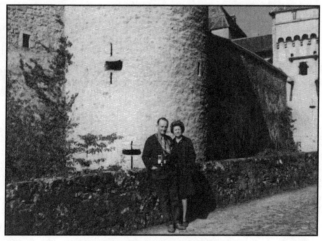

*Mack and Alma at Prison of Chillon
in Switzerland.*

Later Trips

I kept the "H-Stands for Heart Disease" article to use if I ever wanted to initiate a trip; that proved unnecessary.

We have visited all of our 50 states with the exception of Oklahoma.

We have visited:

Canada—from coast to coast.

Mexico—north to south—also Caucun and Tijuana.

South America (Venezuela)

Europe—five trips, four in a rented car.

Asia (1975) a month's trip to Japan, Taiwan, Thailand, Singapore, Indonesia, Kuala Lumpur and Hong Kong.

Africa—Tangier, Rabat and Casablanca

4 Caribbean cruises and a cruise to Alaska.

China? No. We saw China—could have reached through the fence an touched it, but just as God had allowed Moses to view Canaan but forbade entrance, we, too, were not permitted to enter China.

Back in Time:

Changes and events the doctor has seen

As our twentieth century draws to a close it is interesting to reflect upon changes and events observed by my husband, who has lived over 9/10 of the century and 43% of our nation's history.

He saw the change from the horse or mule-drawn vehicles to tractors and combines. He has seen us progress from airplanes to jets, to rockets, space flights and a man on the moon. He saw Halley's Comet in 1910. He remembers the sinking of the *Titanic*.

He can testify of World War I, World War II, the Korean War, and our intervention in Vietnam and the Gulf War.

He saw the rise and fall of Communism.

He recalls the assassination of President John F. Kennedy, civil rights leader Martin Luther King Jr., and Attorney General Robert Kennedy.

He remembers the attempted assassination of President Ronald Reagan and Pope Paul.

Mack endured the Depression beginning in 1929 and the recessions 1949, 1980 and 1982.

He has seen the introduction of the radio, television, and computer.

He endorsed the prohibition of alcoholic beverages, then saw the repeal of the amendment.

He remembers one of the outstanding achievements in 1920 when women won the right to vote, after our nation was a century and a half old.

He welcomed the passage of the Civil Rights Act of 1957 and 1964.

In the field of medicine, Mack has seen the advent of insulin, the "miracle" antibiotic drugs, electrocardiograms, x-rays, and blood banks.

He has welcomed the eradication of polio, diphtheria, typhoid and smallpox. He has seen vaccines developed for tetanus, rabies, measles, whooping cough, mumps, diphtheria and chicken pox.

With the development of computers and scanners one can now find the proverbial needle in the diagnostic haystack.

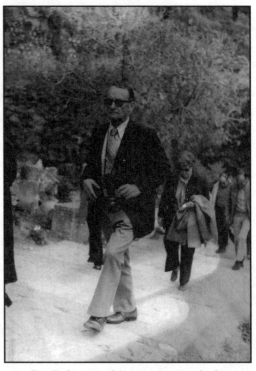

Dr. Roberts on his way to consult the Oracle of Delphi (Greece).

Crutches and braces have been replaced by a wide assortment of new hips, new knees, new elbows, and new shoulders. Perhaps the most amazing innovation of all has been the organ transplant, including the heart. Since 1970 in our country, death from heart attacks has dropped 40%.

Modern medicine has contributed greatly to the quality of life as well as longevity. The doctor has seen life expectancy in America increase from 47 years in 1903 to 75.4 years presently.

There are 52,000 centenarians in America today, twelve times more than in 1965.

His Profession
and Modern Medicine

*"No physician, insofar as he is a physician, considers his own good
in what he prescribes, but the good of the patient; for the true
physician is also a ruler having the human body as a subject,
and is not a mere moneymaker."*
– Plato

For nine decades Dr. Mack Roberts has been an eyewitness of the miracles of modern medicine. Today's doctors prolong our lives in spite of the fact that we abuse our bodies by eating improperly, not exercising enough, doing dope, continuing to puff away at cigarettes and fill emergency rooms with gunshot victims.

Our previously low medical costs have skyrocketed. This has been brought about by the bureaucratization of medical care by state and federal governments, health corporations, health insurance companies, and company owned hospitals.

Doctors are disenchanted with rules and regulations that suffocate them with paperwork and rob them of their independence.

These medical corporations, operating with big business expertise, have about replaced the solo practitioner.

More and more doctors are forced to become salaried employees of managed care networks. They work for the company that owns the hospital rather than for the patient. Many doctors are steered to use the cheapest drugs available often at a risk to the patient.

It is the patient who must pay for many high costs that never enhance the quality of care. Though these institutions deal in bodies, there is sometimes a need to treat the soul.

For the older doctor who has known the joys of being an intimate part of people's lives through respect, caring and understanding, present-day practices cause much frustration. In Mack's case the patient-doctor relationship has become a friendship bond.

We know this association is many times as important as scientific testing. Ordinary complaints can be treated without the extravagant costs of submitting to CAT-scans, x-rays and blood sedimentation tests. Doctors know how to check the pulse without having to make an electrocardiogram. Someone has said many doctors today are more interested in "coining" than "caring."

The medical profession, as other professions, has always had its extortioners. There is an old saying, "Preachers, lawyers, physicians, and buzzard eggs, there's more hatched than come to perfection."

Most doctors will say that the true reward comes from the patient rather than the paychecks.

I know there are exceptions, but I question the wisdom of requiring the elderly or chronically ill to "take up his or her bed and walk"—be transported by ambulance to the doctor's office, instead of the doctor calling on the sick one. If that is "progress" I have the wrong conception of the word.

Dr. Roberts didn't mind God looking over his shoulder, but he found it disgusting with the government, health corporations, etc., calling the calls.

It was an insult for a doctor who has gone through the rigors of medical school and who has had so many years of experience to have to consult some secretary in a distant city for permission to enter a patient into the hospital.

Malpractice suits are as common as detailed descriptions of patients' ailments in the waiting room. Dr. Roberts has no malpractice insurance except his <u>conscience</u>. Malpractice suits for anything and everything remind me of a cartoon in which a mother reads to her child:

> *Jack and Jill*
> *Went up the hill*
> *To fetch a pail of water*
> *Jack fell down and broke his crown*
> *And Jill came tumbling after.*

"Do you suppose they can get a good lawyer?" the child asks.

Dr. Roberts questions our future when a patient will be seen by technicians, then a doctor makes his diagnosis and recommendations from a computer.

Dr. Roberts likes to maintain his medical license. This requires sixty hours of Continuing Education every three years. In July 1996, the doctor completed his requirement at the North Carolina Academy of Family Practice Conference in South Carolina. Over three hundred doctors attended the meeting.

When the head of the seminar learned Mack had practiced sixty-one years and was ninety-three years old, he introduced him to the assembled doctors. Since the average practitioner is now retiring at the age of fifty-five, Dr. Roberts was held up as an inspiration for the doctors. They awarded him a certificate of merit and gave him a book. They also asked him to highlight his career.

The Man and His Philosophy

To bless the weary ones that yearn
For help and comfort every day
For there be such along the way
I SHALL NOT PASS THIS WAY AGAIN.
    –Eva Rose York

What kind of psychic baggage does Dr. Roberts carry? None that he ever divulged. Though in contact daily with conflicting emotions of grief and joy, fear, relief—death, he is known for his equanimity. If you asked him his philosophy, he would say, "Just sit level in the saddle."

He echoed the sentiment of the old gardener who said, "When I sets, I sets loose; when I works, I works hard; when I goes to bed, I sleeps."

Mack lives on the sunny side of life. As someone has said, he dispenses a tranquilizer with no side effects—laughter and lightheartedness.

He is very busy, but it is not his nature to hurry. He can rise at any hour, sleep at any hour or not sleep nor eat for hours. I coveted this gift, but there was no way I could follow suit.

"The doctor is in the business to be bothered," he reasoned, commenting on house calls in the middle of the night. "People don't get sick just during the day."

He is a gregarious person, though not a loquacious one. I found he had greater rapport with the female sex than the male sex.

Though he had no associates, he never practiced alone. He relied on God's help. "I dressed his wounds and God healed him," he would quickly acknowledge.

He enjoyed making house calls, particularly out in the country, to escape the confinement of the office.

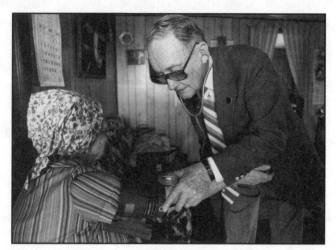

A house call.

A lover of nature, the doctor carried a spade and box to get a start of wild flowers. He also carried a camera. On a trip out west, he photographed every waterfall we saw from Kentucky to California.

Mack put squirrel houses in trees for our squirrels on the creek. Those little creatures, wearing their furry pajamas, traveled our elevated highways (deck railings) carrying hickory nuts and walnuts.

As the patients who came to our house may remember, the doctor had the birds on welfare, though he observed when the weather cleared, the birds elected to make it on their own.

Mack had a running game with the squirrels. Though he fed them, too, he tried to prevent them from robbing the bird feed-ers. One day I found a sign on the bird feeder. "Squirrels Keep Out." The squirrels outwitted the doctor.

Mack had the reputation of being hard on drunks. He felt drunkenness was a self-inflicted sickness. He repeatedly asked drunks where they went to church. But his love for the handicapped and mentally retarded was commendable. "I know," he said, "their parents love them more than if they were not handicapped."

He is everything but an alarmist, which I consider laudable in any physician.

The man could be completely rattled if stopped by a cop in a routine driver's license check. He couldn't find the requested driver's license in ten minutes. Yet, a person would come in who had been in a fight with a chain saw, and Mack would hemstitch on him an hour or more, humming as he worked. He was in his element.

His suturing was better than his handwriting, which re-sembled where a chicken had scratched in the soil for bugs.

Many times I cringed when I saw him touch a wound or skin eruption. "Touching" was part of his manner. I'm sure that patients need to be touched—many lack human contact for a number of reasons. Today, instead of "touching,"there is more likely the reading of signals from a machine or the practice of telemedicine that stretches the limits of bedside manner.

The doctor served as father-confessor to many patients. It gave them great relief to tell him of financial woes; demanding, ungrateful, disobedient children; unfaithful spouses; even to confess their own infidelities. They called them "affairs"—then in *sotto voce* they said, "Doc, could you give me a shot of peni-cillin?"

Their physician listens. No details are too intimate to tell him. Sometimes he wondered if the patient confessed or bragged!

He said he knew enough scandal to put half the county in the penitentiary if he had told it.

God blessed Mack with good health. Much has been said recently concerning emotions and health, laughter and medicine, mind and body.

I think Dr. Roberts subconsciously practiced what many modern day thinkers advocate as mind/body medicine, not only in his work but also personally.

He thought it necessary to understand the patient within family and community context. This is hardly the concept in many managed, present-day practices in which the doctor treats the chart rather than the whole person. Mack greeted his patients with familiarity. He knew their names and their children and grandchildren.

Mack does not like to read or watch anything sad, dirty or negative. If a movie takes a bad turn, he leaves it. He turns off the radio or television when ball games are too close. He focuses on the good things.

Is he not following the Apostle Paul's admonition in Philippians 4:8? "Whatsoever things are true, whatsoever things are honest, whatsoever things are just, whatsoever things are pure, whatsoever things are lovely, whatsoever things are of good report; if there be any virtue, if there be any praise, think on these things."

Worry is not in my spouse's curriculum. After he himself had had surgery for bladder cancer nine years ago, he recently told a friend, "I didn't worry about it."

She, who had had cancer diagnosed, said, "Dr. Roberts, I want to touch you."

I ceased to be surprised that the doctor so good-naturedly accepted patient interruptions at such undesirable times as when we watched the first rockets take off in the Gulf War, or the final seconds in the Kentucky Derby. On Christmas mornings we always had a holdup in gift opening, "while Daddy sees a patient."

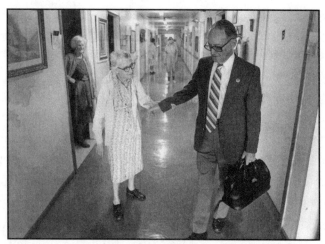

Dr. Roberts greeting patients on Nursing Home round.

When we partied, celebrating Mack's 80th birthday, we had patients come for help; he saw them.

Always he worked on Saturdays—that universal pay day. "I'll pay you Saturday," he had heard all week. "They didn't say which Saturday," he quipped.

For all his lack of assertiveness, he was no pushover.

One sub-zero night about 9:00 p.m., a young man knocked on our door and wanted the doctor to deliver a baby for him. He lived about twelve miles out of town. His house sat at the head of a hollow. The creek became the road the last mile.

Since the fellow already owed my husband for delivering three babies, the doctor could think of many things he would rather do than travel over ice-glazed roads to deliver another free baby for him.

"I've got the money this time, Doc," he said.

When Mack arrived at the cabin, a small fire burned in the fireplace, but to get to his patient's bedroom, he had to climb a ladder. Her room was unheated. The temperature on the inside of the room was comparable to the outside temperature.

The baby arrived soon. The doctor remembers that steam rose off the baby in the frigid room.

After Mack took care of mother and baby, he descended the ladder, warmed himself before the fire, put on his overcoat, hat and gloves, and was ready to go home.

The father-in-law came in and handed Mack a ten dollar bill. "Here is your money," he said. (The price for delivering a baby then was twenty-five dollars.)

The doctor took off his coat, hat and gloves and sat down in a chair. He said, "This fellow already owes me for delivering three babies. He told me he had the money this time. I'm going to sit right here until I get my money."

The father-in-law went back into another room and returned with the fifteen dollars.

The doctor again put on his coat, hat and gloves and headed for home.

Yes, my husband, like the rest of us, had his shortcomings. I'll deal with them later.

His only visible passion is collecting *objets d'art*, figurines, particularly porcelain, crystal, china—anything found in the china section of a department store or antique shop. When I lose him while shopping, and I always do, I know where to search for him.

He knows the joy of generosity. He is an humble man.

He has nursed his first generation into old age and delivered two more generations. Indeed, he saw some from womb to tomb. He never deserted his patients after they became housebound. "Sometimes," he says, "the home situation is mainly what is wrong with them. Besides, look at my fringe benefits."

He appears to forget that people owe him. After his retirement three people looked him up to see how much they owed. Two have paid. He has thousands of dollars of indebtedness on his books. He says he has sent out no more than 50 statements in his life.

My husband is the most forgiving person I have ever known. He refuses to harbor malice.

His Shortcomings

Yes, the doctor has feet of clay, also. Right off, I can think of two imperfections: He is guilty of <u>procrastination</u>. In fact, he is chief of procrastinators—not in his medical work, but otherwise.

The man readily puts off until tomorrow what does not <u>have to be done today</u>. About once a year he says, "What do you want done around here? I have a smart spell on."

Whether or not you consider it a weakness, I think my mate is <u>too trusting</u> in mankind. I know that out there are some impostors and rogues who take advantage of good men.

President Ronald Reagan said it best. "Trust everybody—but cut the cards."

His Love for Poetry

Though Mack found the memorization of poetry distasteful in his early years, poetry has remained with him. When he goes outside on a perfect April morning he quotes:

> *The year's at the spring*
> *And the day's at the morn;*
> *Morning's at seven;*
> *The hillside's dew-pearled;*
> *The lark's on the wing;*
> *The snail's on the thorn;*
> *God's in his heaven —*
> *All's right with the world!*
>
> Robert Browning

Another poem he often quoted is Longfellow's "The Arrow and the Song":

> *The Arrow and the Song*
> *I shot an arrow into the air,*
> *It fell to earth, I knew not where;*
> *For so swiftly it flew, the sight*
> *Could not follow in its flight.*
>
> *I breathed a song into the air,*
> *It fell to earth, I knew not where;*
> *For who has sight so keen and strong,*
> *That it can follow the flight of song?*

Long, long, afterwards, in an oak
I found the arrow, still unbroke;
And the song, from beginning to end,
I found again in the heart of a friend.

A childhood poem surfaces when he sees a brown thrush.

There's a merry brown thrush sitting up in a tree,
"He's singing to me! He's singing to me!"
"And what does he say, little girl, little boy?"
"Oh the world's running over with joy!
Don't you hear? Don't you see?
Hush! Look! In my tree
I'm as happy as happy can be!"
And the brown thrush keeps singing, "A nest do you see,
And five eggs hid in a juniper tree?
Don't meddle, don't touch! Little girl, Little boy,
Or the world will lose some of its joy!
Now I'm glad! Now I'm free!
And I always will be
If you never bring sorrows to me."
So the merry brown thrush sings away in the tree,
To you and to me, to you and to me,
And he sings all the day, little girl, little boy,
"Oh the is world running over with joy
But long it won't be
Don't you know? Don't you see?
Unless we're as good as can be."

Lucy Larcom (1826-1893)

Alma Roberts

Mack sits patiently and attentively through a rousing business meeting with the following quotation running through his mind.

> *A Wise Old Owl*
> *A wise old owl lived in an oak;*
> *The more he saw the less he spoke;*
> *The less he spoke the more he heard;*
> *Why can't we all be like that bird?*

Our travels seem to bring his poetry to mind repeatedly. In England when he viewed our first castle in the distance, he quoted:

> *The splendor falls on castle walls*
> *And snowy summits old in story:*
> *The long light shakes across the lakes*
> *And the wild cataract leaps in glory.*
> *Blow, bugle, blow, set the wild echoes flying,*
> *Blow, bugle, answer; echoes, dying, dying, dying.*
> Alfred Tennyson (1802-92)

At the seaside he recites from Tennyson:

> *Break, break, break*
> *On thy cold gray stones, O sea!*
> *And I would that my tongue could utter*
> *The thoughts that arise in me.*

When our French guide escorted us across the battlements of the fort in the double-walled city of Carcassonne in France, Mack began to quote:

> *How old I am! I'm sixty years!*
> *I have worked hard all my life;*
> *Yet, patient as my life has been,*
> *One dearest sight I have not seen*
> *It almost seems a wrong;*
> *A dream I had when I was young,*
> *Alas, our dreams they come not true!*
> *I hoped to see fair CARCASSONNE*
> *That lovely city CARCASSONNE.*

Mack quoted at length from the seven stanza poem. Madame said, "That poem is in this pamphlet I will give you."

After spending several days in Ireland, Mack, Helen, our son-in-law Patrick Deese, and I left Dublin and crossed the Irish Sea by ferry for Liverpool, England. We were headed for the magical country of Wales. I, particularly, wished to visit again the River Dee near Llangollen. It is without a doubt the prettiest river I have ever seen.

I remember it was Sunday and an English holiday when we had left Liverpool in our rented car. Everyone was going to the beach.

Traffic came to a halt on an incline. An angry motorist from behind us rapped on our car window and said to our driver, Pat, "You hit me—you rolled back and hit me."

"Did we hit you? I didn't know we hit you. I'm sorry," our soft-spoken Alabamian son-in-law said. "Oh, forget it," said the

Englishman and returned to his car. "A soft answer turneth away wrath" (Proverbs 15:1).

When we neared Conwy, Wales, Conwy Castle gleamed brightly from afar. The eight towers, each with walls 15 feet thick, rose to a height of 70 feet. We toured the medieval castle. I had never heard of Conwy (Conway). The name "Conwy" brought to Mack's mind Wordsworth's "We Are Seven," a poem he had memorized in part, in elementary school. He recited a part of the poem:

> *A simple little child*
> *That lightly draws its breath*
> *And feels its life in every limb*
> *What should it know of death?*
>
> *I met a little cottage girl,*
> *She was eight years old, she said;*
> *Her hair was thick with many a curl*
> *That clustered round her head.*
>
> *She had a rustic, woodland air.*
> *And she was wildly clad:*
> *Her eyes were fair, and very fair; -*
> *Her beauty made me glad.*
>
> *"Sisters and brothers, little maid*
> *How many may you be?"*
> *"How many? Seven in all," she said*
> *And wondering looked at me.*

> *"And where are they, I pray you tell?"*
> *She answered, "Seven are we;*
> *And two of us at Conway dwell,*
> *And two are gone to sea..."*

Later when we visited the River Dee, Mack began to recite from Charles Kingsley's tragic poem, "The Sands O'Dee"

> *"Oh, Mary, go and call the cattle home,*
> *And call the cattle home,*
> *And call the cattle home,*
> *Across the sands O'Dee!"*
> *The western wind was wild and dank with foam,*
> *And all alone went she.*

Our son-in-law said his family reportedly came from the River Dee area and were called "Deese" for that reason.

After I had lost two brothers in a car accident Mack bought me a book of poetry. He marked one poem, "Read this":

> *If you should go before me, dear, walk slowly,*
> *Down the ways of death, well-worn and wide,*
> *For I would want to overtake you quickly*
> *And seek the journey's ending by your side.*

> *I would be so forlorn not to descry you*
> *Down some shining high road where I came;*
> *Walk slowly, dear, and often look behind you*
> *And pause to hear if someone calls your name.*

The Grandchildren Speak

Grandfather

School assignment written by Mack Drake (age 13)

A hat, a medicine bag, a prescription pad, a stethoscope, and a Jeep Wagoneer. Kind, thoughtful, caring, brilliant, humble. All of these things describe one person and one person only in Wayne County. That person would be Dr. Mack Roberts. Not many other doctors I know have practiced medicine for 61 years. Not many doctors have delivered a baby for as low as $25.00. To me, he is a grandfather and a friend. He has delivered over 4,200 babies in his life, treated millions of colds, and stitched up thousands of cuts.

Dr. Roberts is no ordinary doctor. If he were eating supper and a sick patient came to his home, he did not make them wait—he treated them right then. Midnight house calls were not unusual. On the way to a sick patient's rural home, he would take his Jeep as far as it would go, then take a horse or mule, or just walk. Here is a story of his devotion to helping others . . . It's midnight, and while most of Wayne County sleeps, a light burns in a window of "Doc's" house. Worried parents have brought a little girl with a high fever. Soon, they have left. Dr. Roberts can possibly get another hour's sleep if he is lucky before he is summoned to the aid of another sick person. Dr. Roberts did not even retire until he was 90 years old!

There is no one characteristic that makes Dr. Roberts so special. His dry wit, his eternal optimism, and his easygoing nature have made him a favorite. I have been very fortunate to have lived all my 13 years next door to this distinguished gentleman. When I was younger, one of my favorite outdoor adventures was for my grandfather to take me "snake hunting" with a .22 rifle. Today, in the hot summers, he and I shoot lizards lying on rocks in the

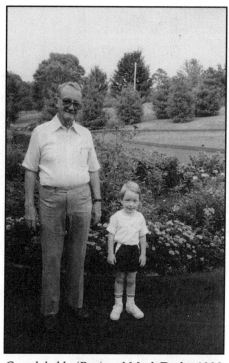

Grand daddy (Pop) and Mack Drake, 1986.
"Lets go snake hunting, Pop."

flower garden. He and I have gotten to be crack shots! His vegetable garden lies along our creek, and it is easier for him at his age to drive his Bravada through the field and down the steep hill than to walk to it. He delights in allowing me to drive him on this bumpy venture, and of course, I am delighted to practice my driving skills.

Perhaps Doc is most known for flowers or his Jeep, but I believe in my heart, that he is best known for his kindness.

Grandaddy

Grandad of Tara, Mark, Aimee and Mack
Lover of family, God and mankind
Who feels fulfilled when helping others, joy from family,
And happiness from a robin's song
Who fears disharmony in family, missing an afternoon nap,
And being unable to help others
Who would like to see morality among all,
all of his family together
And spring days on the creek
Resident of Monticello, Kentucky
Roberts

Aimee Looney Touchstone

Pop Remembers

School assignment by Mack Drake (age 13)

When I recently asked my ninety-three-year-old grandfather what was an occurrence that most stood out in his mind, he responded with three answers. Let me relay these events to you today.

The first event he recalled took place in 1912. This event was the sinking of the R.M.S. *Titanic.* My grandfather recalled much discussion between friends and neighbors about the ship that was declared "unsinkable." He remembers it was on its maiden voyage from Southampton, England, to New York. For a time, the ship was really gossiped about among Monticello residents. He then recounted what was said to have happened on the *Titanic's* doomsday. He remembered many of the names of rich

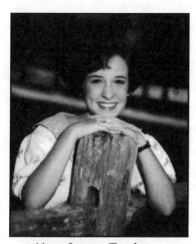

Aimee Looney Touchstone graduated Summa Cum Laude from David Lipscomb University. She teaches Kindergarten in Huntsville, Alabama.

people that died when it sank. These names included Colonel Archibald Butt, a retired colonel, and John Jacob Astor, a millionaire. Abijah Burnett, a Monticello citizen, remarked, "Archibald Butt—a thoroughbred Roman Catholic." Dr. Roberts, my grandfather, also recalled what was said to have sunk the ship. "Apparently, the 'unsinkable' ship ignored warnings of an ice field ahead and struck an iceberg, damaging the hull at the bow of the ship." He also remembered there not being enough lifeboats to carry all passengers on the ship. He recalled all of the women and children being loaded first. He found out the terrible news while reading the newspaper. There were no telephones or radios at his home. He was nine at the time, and lived in Oil Valley—seven miles east of Monticello.

The second event occurred in 1918, toward the end of World War One. My grandfather, along with his brothers and father were shucking corn on their farm when they heard the sawmill whistles all start to blow in Monticello at an unusual time. They had been previously told that on that day, the Armistice was to be signed in the Palace of Versailles in France. That is the treaty that brought World War One to an end. Germany and the Kaiser were defeated! (My grandfather had a mule at this time named Kaiser Wilhelm!) Everyone in my grandfather's family started celebrating and rejoicing because of two reasons. One, the war was over, and two, his brother that was to be drafted the next day, would not have to go fight!

Later on that day, they found out it was a false alarm—the Armistice had not been signed that day as planned! The next day, as everyone went about their chores sadly, on the eleventh month, the eleventh day, the eleventh hour, 1918, the whistles went off again. This time, they could rejoice! It was the real thing!

The third event my grandfather recalled was not on an international, national, or even state level. It took place right here in Wayne County, around 1910-1912. That event was when he saw the first car in Monticello. My grandfather was riding behind his father on a horse on their way to church. His brothers were also riding horses, when they heard an "awful racket" coming toward them. They soon spied the source of this sound—an automobile! The man in the car knew that their horses could have never seen a car before, so the man turned off and stopped his car and led my grandfather's horses past his car. This was the first car my grandfather ever saw. "Horses were literally scared to death of automobiles—they would run off," stated my grandfather. An oil man, Harry Mooney, owned this first car. Dr. Gamblin had an early car with a sprocket chain on the outside like a bicycle. Some neighbor kids of my grandfather rode home in a car from school and were promptly whipped by their father because cars were considered "unsafe"!

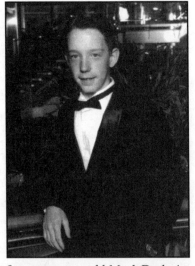

Seventeen-year-old Mack Drake is a veteran traveler, an avid reader, a water sports enthusiast, and an expert pianist. The senior at Monticello High School maintains a 4.0 GPA.

They say that in every one's life there are some special events that stand out more than anything, and that person remembers where he was and what he was doing when these events occurred. These have been three events that stand out in the early life of my grandfather.

Lessons on Life from Granddaddy

By Tara Looney Swafford

When I was given the opportunity to write about my Granddaddy, two things immediately came to mind. While there are many remarkable characteristics about my grandfather, there are two that I treasure most: his genuine devotion to people and his pervasively optimistic view of life.

His devotion to his patients was extraordinary. I can remember countless family gatherings that were interrupted by calls and visits from patients. It was rare that Christmas Day went by without Granddaddy being taken away to care for one of his patients. The rest of the family was always a bit annoyed that our gathering was being interrupted, but Granddaddy never hesitated to help whatever patient was in need at the time—even if it meant leaving in the middle of Mamommy's wonderful Christmas dinner.

Granddaddy never seemed to get a day's rest from the demands of his patients. I remember when as kids my brother, sister and I would visit Monticello, Granddaddy started keeping a collection of all the fees he earned from house calls during our visit. He would then split the total among the three of us (and later the four of us when little Mack arrived; Granddaddy was always careful about treating everyone equally). So, we, of course, became keenly interested in the arrival of patients and

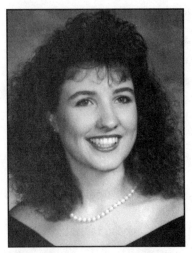

Tara Looney Swafford graduated Summa Cum Laude from Case Western Reserve Law School. She practices law in Nashville, Tennessee.

the house calls. It turned what used to be our annoyance at the interruptions into a game to see how many patients Granddaddy could see during our visit. As I recall, no single patient ever netted over $15-$20; and, frequently, $5 was the most received. I wonder now how many times Granddaddy just kicked in money of his own after visits so we wouldn't be disappointed when he finished with his patients. I am also amazed now when I recall that $150-$200 was the average intake for a three to a four-day span that included numerous patients. Granddaddy truly gave a generous amount of time, expertise, and kindness with little expectation for remuneration.

I even had the honor of being a patient of Granddaddy's. In second grade, I cut my chin in a bike wreck and had to have stitches. Granddaddy came all the way to Paris, Tennessee, to assist in taking the stitches out, but he first demonstrated on my doll to show how easy it would be. Needless to say, I was much more at ease knowing Granddaddy was taking care of me.

Undoubtedly, the greatest reason for the respect and love I have for my grandfather is his amazing outlook on life. It is hard for anyone to describe, much less understand, how he truly never has a derogatory comment to say about anyone or anything and can always find something positive or humorous to say whatever the situation. I don't know the explanation for his constantly positive demeanor, but I can speculate that his faith in God and his love for others form the root of true self-contentment that is manifested in the way he treats others and lives life.

Whatever the reason, I firmly believe that Granddaddy's attitude is the primary reason for his incredibly long, happy and productive life. I feel truly blessed to have had a grandfather that has taught me to care for others, no matter who they are, and that human beings do have the capability to be uplifting and content in any given circumstance. This world would be a much better place if we could all follow his example. I am sure that Monticello, Kentucky, has greatly benefited from it. I know my family has.

Mark Roberts Looney's Application to Medical School

The twin questions of what a person is and why he is what he is have always intrigued me. As I approach the major decision time in my life, these questions provide more than an intellectual curiosity.

My father is a lawyer and my older sister is in law school, but I could not imagine a more boring use of my time. My paternal grandparents own a funeral home where I have spent many interesting hours. Although I have learned important lessons through my expo-

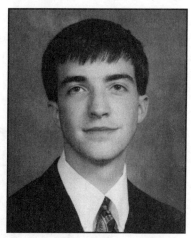

Mark Roberts Looney, M.D., graduated from the University of Tennessee Medical School with a 4.0 average and was selected for membership in Alpha Omega Alpha. He is now in his 3rd year of residency at the University of California at San Francisco.

sure to death, the profession is not in my immediate future. My undergraduate education helped pinpoint the passion I have for science, but my professional future remained nebulous at best. I was still convinced that the proper development of my mind and the traits I inherited would answer the question of who I am and what I am to become.

My ultimate decision to pursue a medical career has been greatly influenced by my maternal grandfather. The admiration I have for the medical field has grown out of my relationship with him. He and I share the same birthday, and on July 24 he will be 90 years old. He practiced medicine in a small Southeastern Kentucky community until one month ago when he finally retired. He is "Doc" to all who know him, rich and poor, powerful and disadvantaged, and the old and young. It appears he was born to be a doctor in the hills of the home he never left. I believe a good part of him is in me, and after a summer of changing the diapers of the incontinent, bathing the sick and injured, and seeing the healing art where it meets the people, I can not think of anything else God put me here to do.

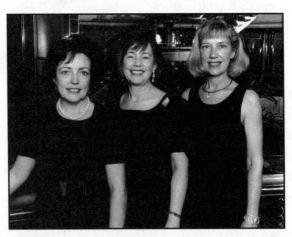

Our three daughters in 1997 on an Alaskan cruise taken by the whole family. Ann (left), Helen (center), Marilyn (right).

Lineage

And sometimes, when I have become
A quiet portrait on the wall,
Will you, my far descendant,
Stop to think of me at all?

Suppose your hands are shaped like mine —
You have my nitwit sense of fun —
Will there be one to tell you so, there,
When my days are done?

If you love books, and fires and songs,
And slipper moons on lilac skies,
Toss me a look of shared delight
From those, my own blue eyes.

For there is kinship in a curl,
And keepsake in a spoken name,
And wine of life may yet be poured
By hands within a frame.

Author Unknown

Back Then

Dr. Roberts's patients were never taken from their beds and loaded into an ambulance and delivered to his office. The doctor went to see them. He says, "In the 1930s, 40s and even into the 50s, the first hurdle in making a house call was not making the correct diagnosis but in reaching the patient."

Most of our local streams had no bridges. They were forded at a shallow place by car, Jeep—or horse or crossed by footlog.

To reach the Panhandle area of our county, across the Cumberland River, one crossed in a dinky, community ferry if a car was taken. If the car were to be abandoned, he would blow the horn and an acquaintance would come down to the river and "set Doc across" in a skiff. Doc would then walk or ride a horse or mule to his destination. Those crossings occurred at nighttime as well as during daytime. The people who lived on the river were wonderful to Mack. He hasn't forgotten them.

He tells of one person, Mr. Will Scott, who was afraid for him to go alone into certain areas. Moonshiners were known to shoot farmers off mowing machines in some of those rough communities. He feared Mack might be mistaken for a "revenoor." Mr. Scott had his son accompany Mack when he called on the Ard School as Health Officer.

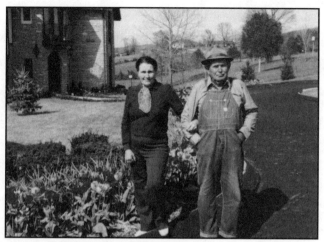

Our dear friends, Laura and Charlie Morgan.

Remembered Accolades

After the doctor's retirement a former patient, father of thirteen, came into his office at the bank.

Former patient: "You don't know me, do you, Doc?"

Doc: "Yes, I know you."

Former patient: "Doc, you are the wonderfulest man that's ever been in this county."

Nursing Home patient: "Dr. Roberts's head is not big enough to hold all the stars he'll have in his crown."

Speaker: "How's Doc?"

"He's fine."

Speaker: "There'll never be another one like him. He is the only doctor I ever had, 'cept when I was in the army."

A young mother comes to our front door. She has a seven-week angel in her carrier—a beautiful child. She is very sick.

"They kept her a whole week at University Hospital. I didn't find out anything. Everyone tells me to take her to Dr. Roberts; he knows what he's doing."

Patient: "I told my husband if I just had one wish I'd wish for Dr. Roberts to be young again." That is the kindest statement I have heard anyone say about my husband.

WAVE Television of Louisville arranged to come to Monticello to do a program on the doctor. We invited the fellows out for lunch at the Captain's Table of the Anchor Motel.

We arrived at the restaurant before our guests.

"Hey, Doc," a local black person hailed the doctor. "There were some guys in here this morning from a Louisville television station, interviewing everybody about you. I told 'em you'd delivered a bunch of kids for me and of course Doc never got anything out of it."

The ultimate compliment is paid when a patient goes to a "big city" to see a specialist, returns home, and calls Dr. Roberts to ask him if it's all right to take the medicine the doctor prescribed.

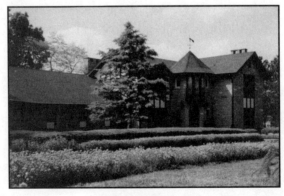

The house that Mack and Alma built.

Reminiscence

Today when we travel roads the doctor traversed so often, he reminisces. There is a story at nearly every house we pass—memories drifting through his mind as easily as the wind riffles the dead leaves across the road.

He points to a house on Morris Hill. "There's where I delivered twins. When I asked for diapers, the mother said, 'There was a diaper around here somewhere, but I don't know where.'"

At Mill Springs he indicates a house on a hilltop. "I delivered a baby there. The father wasn't at home. As I was leaving, I saw him coming around the ridge. He called to see what had happened."

"You have twins," I joked.

"What did you say?"

"You have twins."

"Hell fire!"

"There," Mack nods to a house by the side of the road in McCreary County, "I waited for the arrival of a baby. The expectant mother wouldn't get into bed—she walked continually. As her pains increased, I urged her to go to bed. She ignored my warning.

"'Spat!' The baby's head hit the floor. I thought the fall had probably killed it, but the baby appeared to be all right."

The doctor refers to a house in One-Eye Hollow. "I was there to deliver a baby. Rats as big as cats ran across the room."

He cites a house on the Cooper Road. "Dr. C. B. Rankin had been there all day on a case of obstetrics. Late in the afternoon, he called for me to come help him. 'And bring some chewing gum and cigars,' he said."

At a place in Owl Town he said, "I remember coming out here one snowy night. I rode a red mule part of the way. I delivered a baby and collected ten dollars. I was glad to get it." It had been during the years of his early practice.

In Sheep Lot he cites a home. "An old woman lived there with a houseful of cats. The smell was sickening," the doctor said. He solved his problem by carrying a spray can of deodorant in his bag. "Every time my patient turned her head, I'd spray a whiff of deodorizer."

We pass a nursing home—"Bill (a patient there) used to give himself insulin shots through his overalls."

At Rogers' Grove the doctor points to a house where a gracious black man lived who always asked the doctor when he entered the house, "Doctor, can I rest your hat?"

We are driving through the Concord community. "One rainy night," the doctor said, "I drove to here, then walked by lantern light over the hill to see an old gentleman. He paid me with a ten dollar gold bill." The doctor still has the gold bill.

On York Trail, near Eadsville, the doctor said, "Over there I walked through a muddy field one night to deliver a baby. I remember five small children were bedded in one bed."

A Special Memory

One fine April day my husband calls me from his office and asks me to accompany him on a house call out in the country.

We drive south about twelve miles, take a left off our graveled road and proceed up a dirt road that coils beside a tum-

bling creek. We follow that stream up a hill until our road be-
comes a wagon trail.

Our trusty Jeep climbs slowly over the bumpy way that leads
us into a woods wearing a green haze. I roll my window down
to smell the fresh air and find the woodland a-twitter with
bird song.

This is the magical season. Magenta beaded redbuds flaunt
their beauty at the edge of the timber. Those flowers will be
replaced by heart-shaped leaves as red as a newborn baby.

On some varieties of trees, buds are just beginning to swell.
Dogwoods appear to be cautiously awaiting the signal to burst
into flower and fruition. I think one hot day or even a clap of
thunder could set off the whole works. We can almost hear the
growth of spring.

A cardinal flashes by. We cross a brook.

"Stop," I say. Mack, knowing my delight in brooks, water-
falls and woods, asks no questions. He likes them too. He stops
the car. There is something about "being in it"—making contact
with nature.

We get out of the car and inhale the earthy smell mingled
with the tingling aroma of the pines. April had set up house-
keeping right here.

I am captivated by the little stream. The water spouts, spurts
and spills over rocks. What is its hurry? Is it akin to society? I
bend to test the water. It is cold.

Fiddlehead ferns emerging from last season's dead foliage
fringe the soggy banks of the branch. They are plentiful.

"Let's gather some for supper," I suggest. I had prepared
them before. We had first eaten them in Nova Scotia. Mack pro-
duces his pocket knife. I find an empty plastic bag in the back
of the Jeep. We pick enough for a mess. Fiddleheads and corn
cakes. I could almost taste them.

Trees are all around us: pines, hickories, stately poplars and lichened oaks. Sun and shadow play through their leafless branches as they sway in the gentle breeze. Beech trees retain last year's leaves. Their pale and crisp leaves rustle on their twigs. The trees have smooth gray bark—the kind lovers carve their initials on.

We walk on springy pine needles to the northeastern slope. Colonies of trillium and mayapples are blooming. We smell the fragrance of the sweet williams.

I flop down on a soft chestnut log overgrown by mosses. I imbibe the after rain-like woodland fragrance, chew on a sprig of mint, and listen to the mournful, insistent "coo" of a dove.

White flowered bloodroots polka dot the hillside. They are beginning to shed. I see crowsfeet in bloom in company with foamflowers. A couple of jacks-in-the-pulpit try to hide their flower spikes under a hood.

Mack stands with one foot propped on a log, entirely absorbed by I know not what.

"What do those cross strips of wood nailed to the tree trunks mean?" He scratches his head in a quandary and points toward a smattering of trees.

I had not looked beyond my immediate enchantment. We cannot understand the meaning of those pieces of wood attached to the trees.

We note that wildflowers follow the return of the migrant birds, just as birds follow the return of spring.

"Let's go," the doctor says, "I have other calls to make after this one."

In the car again, Mack winds and wends his way by a faint trail through the timberland as if he had been born there. How he found this remote place, I will never know. We pass through too quickly. I could linger in this unhurried place.

We veer to the left to avoid one of the trees with cross pieces. We skirt a fallen branch that has almost blocked our way and follow a wide path out of the woods.

Behold, right in front of us is a sun-splashed meadow of ten or twelve acres defined by a split-rail cedar fence, enclosed by hills and an overhanging pine-topped cliff. Here is a world of its own. We have made a discovery—a little Switzerland!

Three red cows wearing clanking bells graze the upland pasture. They stare at us. There are no trees on this tract. The plot is interlaced with cow paths.

Our trail descends to a Lincoln-vintage log house and barn. I see no evidence of weeds having invaded this domain. I see no signs of "civilization." No beer cans, paper cups or discarded household plunder clutter the landscape.

No chickens, geese or guineas announce our arrival. No dogs run out and yelp at us. Other than the sound of the dove, the "caw, caw, caw" of crows flapping toward the cliff and my racing imagination, I hear nothing. The tranquillity is almost palpable.

A bittersweet vine clambers over the house's mud-daubed stone chimney. A Texas-sized clump of bleeding hearts blooms beside the doorway. I see no other flowers.

An aging bachelor, Odie, and his elderly sister, Sara, sole family survivors, live in this isolated place. With the brother sick abed, the responsibility to see to everything has fallen upon the sister.

After attending the patient, Mack asks Sara about the cross-pieces of wood on the trees we had seen.

The Seth Thomas clock on the mantel ticks loudly while Sara hesitates to answer. At last, she explains there had been mad foxes in the area. She had feared that she, while gathering wood, might be attacked. She had planned her escape route, hoping the crosspieces would serve as a ladder for her to get away from the rabid foxes.

That memory has persisted. Now many years later, every time I see bleeding hearts my thoughts return to what we refer to as the "fox woman's place."

The family of two is gone. I am sure that little Eden has reverted to wilderness.

How I wish I could have known them, Odie and Sara. What wisdom they might have imparted to me, those two, who like the psalmist, looked to the hills for help and feasted on manna from heaven.

I wonder: Does the place have a sense of abandonment? Has the old house collapsed? Do foxes still bark and maraud? Do crows still nest on that imposing cliff? Did Sara ever have to flee from a fox by means of her "ladders"?

Are those perennial bleeding hearts still blooming, unseen? Did they bespeak the lives of those two solitary people—that once there was a woman, or a man, who suffered from a broken heart?

Loneliness, they say, is the greatest poverty.

Such was the pay and often the only reward the doctor received for a call.

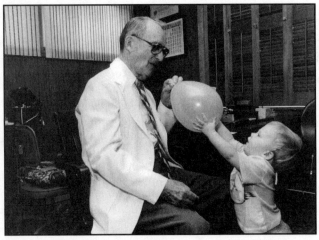

Mutual love—he pleases a child with a balloon.

His Viewpoint

"Every generation of Americans needs to know that freedom consists not in doing what we like, but having the right to do what we ought."
–Pope John Paul

Dr. Roberts looks to the past and bemoans what our nation has lost: strong family ties, close ties to God, safe schools and streets.

We live in a time of implausibility. Low self-esteem is often used as an alibi for violence. The doctor would advise us to concentrate on self-control or discipline rather than self-esteem.

He regrets that we have gone from using no keys for our homes to the necessity for security systems.

Yet, he is pleased to see the diminishing of discrimination, and a great decrease in illiteracy and ill health.

He sees our government as having strayed too far from the moral principles on which our nation was founded. He realizes our salvation is only in a spiritual revival in America.

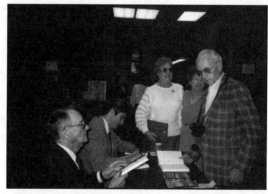

Dr. Howard Wallace Roberts, great-nephew of Dr. Roberts and author of Doc, autographs his book at the Monticello Banking Company, 1987. (standing left to right) Elba Wilhite, Alma Roberts, Shelby Keeton.

To Work or Not to Work

Folks who never do anymore than they get paid for,
never get paid for any more than they do.
–Elbert Hubbard

The Bible indicates there is a time to work—and a time to rest. The Sabbath law, in part, was an example of God saying, "You need a rest." The Mosaic law ordained Sabbaticals that every seventh year the land and vineyards were to remain fallow, and prescribed that there would be celebrated the year of Jubilee, a year-long celebration held every fifty years when land was left fallow.

The doctor grasped that fact slowly.

"Why don't you retire?" he was often asked by a concerned relative.

"I haven't found anything to do I like better," the doctor said.

At a time when working until age sixty-three or sixty-five was once the norm and in recent years when more than one-third of male laborers between fifty-five and sixty years of age disappear from the work force voluntarily or by downsizing, there Dr. Roberts rode full tilt, like a modern-day Don Quixote, battling injury, disease and death—not until age sixty, sixty-five, seventy, seventy-five, eighty, eighty-five, but until age ninety. Over the hill, he seemed to accelerate.

Ready for retirement myself, I protested. "I thought you said you would retire on your birthday."

"I didn't say which birthday," he teased.

Why did he persevere? What motivated him?

1. His love for his work.
2. His continued good health.
3. The obligation he felt to his faithful patients who had for years deplored, "What will we ever do if Doc quits?"
4. The high cost of medical treatment. Though we now had good roads and a good local hospital, our patients complained, "Doc, I can't afford to go to the Emergency Room. The last time I went, it cost so and so." The doctor knew many of them could not afford these charges.
5. His zest for life.

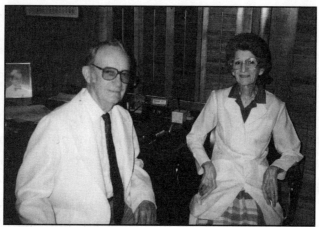

Dr. Mack and cousin Aleta Roberts, for 24 years his receptionist and secretary.

His secret? Not "Do what you like," but "Like what you do."

Years before, I had said, "You've worked fifty years. How about a year of Jubilee?"

"You either practice medicine, or you don't," he said. Of course, he was right.

How I wished Jesus had said, "They also serve, who only stand and wait."

I find in my diary: "I am as fed up with this life as the children of Israel were fed up with manna."

I continued to put my dream of writing on hold.

Eight sabbatical years had passed. Emotionally I packed my bags, but my admiration always prevailed—admiration for the doctor's dedication, his care, his loyalty to his patients—he didn't cop out on them.

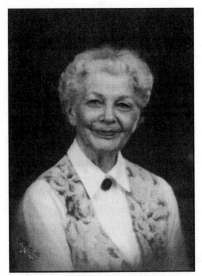

Jo Ann Powell Anderson, a wonderful receptionist for many years.

I reprimanded myself. What a privilege to hold up the hands of one so devoted to the art of healing.

I had in the meantime become older and felt the need for fewer interruptions. Yet, I empathized with our patients who, filled with anxiety, approached me at the grocery and said they had heard "Doc is going to quit."

I still dreamed of my cottage small by a waterfall with neither doorbell, telephone, radio, television nor mail. William Butler Yeats expressed my wish well:

> *And I shall have some peace there, for peace comes dropping slow,*
> *Dropping from the veils of morning to where the cricket sings;*
> *There midnight's all a glimmer, and noon a purple glow,*
> *And evenings full of linnet's wings.*
>
> *The Lake Isle of Innisfree*

The Year of Jubilee:

After Sixty-one Years in the Saddle, the Doctor Dismounts

He warmed both hands before the fire of life.
–Walter Savage Landor

Tales of Dr. Roberts's impending retirement had circulated for twenty-five years. Dr. Roberts retired July 1, 1993.

Why did this nonagenarian **finally** retire?

1. He was fed up with bureaucracy in the medical field.
2. He became disgusted with drug abuse among certain patients.
3. His hearing diminished.
4. A bum knee slowed him perceptibly.
5. He wished to devote more time to the Monticello Banking Company of which he has been president for twenty years and a director for fifty-two years.
6. He wanted to please his wife, who was ready to shout "Brother!" (I had begun to feel frustration to the **nth** degree.)

The doctor will tell you that for the first fifty years, I gave unstintingly to support him in his worthy work. However, in the last few years, the practice of medicine had become tarnished by dope addicts. Our office, as other doctors' offices, had been broken into several times. Our home had been broken into and

I felt an uneasiness that had never before surfaced.

In speaking of his retirement, the doctor said he was like the man who cut off his monkey's tail two inches at a time because he didn't think the monkey could stand it if he cut all of it off at once. The doctor had slowed down gradually.

First, he began to take off Friday afternoons if we left home.

Next, he took off Wednesdays if we left town.

On the doctor's "days off," we were awakened earlier, not by our alarm clock or biological clocks, but by the insistent ringing of the doorbell or telephone by someone who had not wanted to wait his turn in the office. "I'll just wait and catch Doc at home." Or it might be someone who stops to see him on his way to work. Of course, there were always accidents and such.

Our ten-year-old grandson, Mack Drake, who lived next door, put up a sign on the door.

NOTICE:

Dr. Roberts is NOT seeing
Patients today.
Thank you,

CLOSED

The first patient read the sign and, undaunted, rang the doorbell. The doctor hesitated and then admitted him.

I began to wonder—could it be momentum?

But he did **draw the line**.

I went to the laundromat the day of his retirement. Everyone began to tell me how they regretted losing their doctor. One woman said, "Doc saved my life."

A fellow who rides a motorbike around town said, "I don't know what in the world I'll do for a doctor. Doc's always been my doctor. He birthed me."

I went to the grocery store that day. At the checkout counter the retirement was mentioned. A person said, "Doc was the poor man's doctor; he'll treat you if you have the money or not."

Another said, "Mama said Doc Roberts borned me. She said I was a ten dollars baby—yeah, I costed ten dollars. He borned half of Wayne County."

Early the next morning I overheard a phone conversation. A patient from Burnside called. "Doc, I can't get your office atall."

"I've retired."

"You've retired! What will we do, Doc?"

"Well, I'm ninety. I thought it was about time to quit."

"You ninety?"

A couple of days later, a woman who had moved from Wayne County to Somerset, in Pulaski County, called. She had heard Dr. Roberts had retired.

They reminisced.

"You delivered seven of my ten children, Dr. Roberts. You named one of them—John Henry. You took his tonsils out, too. I still owe you, but you said to forget it."

"Yeah, we marked that off," the doctor said.

The woman continued—her daughter had promised to bring her down to see the doctor.

After the retirement announcement, we immediately set out on a Caribbean Cruise, taking as many of our family as could accompany us (seven). We celebrated "Daddy's" ninetieth birthday and retirement. We had a joyful, memorable trip.

We returned home and celebrated the doctor's birthday for a

month with kith and friends. Like wine, he gets better with age.

After we returned from our cruise, the roar of our busy world had begun to subside. There were still callers who refused to believe "Doc has retired."We continue six years later to have callers and phone contacts.

Did we find the change very noticeable? It was like escaping a rainstorm on the interstate by passing under an overpass.

Now was the time to get on with our happily-ever-aftering.

We are told it is important to walk racehorses after a race. The doctor agrees with that principle wholeheartedly. He dared not come to a sudden stop.

Since retirement he goes each morning to his office at the Monticello Banking Company.

From what I hear, much reminiscing goes on in that office. "Doc, do you remember that night I met you down at the creek on a horse and you rode up the holler...?" The doctor usually remembers and can supply details. For **once**, he has time to really visit with friends.

When we travel the country roads, the doctor might stop with some farmers chatting over a fence, and ask some foolish question such as, "Is this the right road to Parnell?" when we are in the wrong part of the county.

"Doc, what are you doing out here?"

My husband doesn't know everyone in the county, but everyone knows him except the very young and newcomers. Because I'm "Doc Roberts's wife," most of them know me, too. Today, a lady at the funeral home, whose name I could not recall, said, "You've answered the door for me many a time."

Did the doctor suffer post-partum depression or withdrawal pains? No!

Sometimes he smiles and says, "Got to work a haircut into my schedule today."

On a snowy night he might say, "This is a good time not to have to go to Owl Town on a mule to deliver a baby."

The phone continued to ring. "He's retired!" I said. I feared I had a note of gladness in my voice, but there was sympathy in my heart for the caller.

"Are you napping too much?" I once asked my husband.

"Rip Van Winkle did pretty well at it," he said.

Then I remember so vividly how he had been disturbed during naptime, probably an average of three times per nap.

Now, in the Indian Summer of life, you will find him in his recliner by the fireside in the winter. There is a stack of reading material including medical journals and the Bible beside him.

On the table top is the phone. A book or the phone is usually in his hand. He watches the news and some sports on television when the contest isn't too close.

In the summertime he fiddles in his garden, portable phone in hip pocket. It has saved him many a trip up the hillside to answer a call. Now, because of a painful knee, he drives over the hill in his Wagoneer. He has tended a vegetable garden every year of our married life until this year.

He continued to answer the door for Halloweeners until recently.

As mentioned earlier, the doctor attends continuing medical education conferences. He has just completed the requirement for 60 hours to maintain his license for three more years.

He continues to operate his farm at Mill Springs.

He is a faithful member of the Elk Spring Valley Baptist Church and is a dedicated member of the Gideon Society.

He travels widely. At his age of ninety-two, we went to South America. He celebrated his ninety-fourth birthday in Alaska.

I find it a heart-lifting experience to accompany the doctor to gatherings and see the reception he receives.

And what did I do after his retirement? I began to live the life I had imagined. I repossessed my husband who had belonged to the people; now he is **mine**.

In the meantime, we had found our sanctuary, in town, on the fifteen-acre property on Elk Creek we have owned for a number of years. Our place had been "sanctified" by General George Patton, who bivouacked here during the days of Troop B and later Troop K, a local cavalry unit of the National Guard.

Our architect hit all the right notes, as far as we are concerned in planning our Tudor style house. With thirteen glass doors and three windows on the creek side of the house we have all the beauty of nature pouring in. Though God created heaven and earth in six days, it took a bit longer , fifteen months, to build our house.

Despite the fact we aren't that far from the "maddening crowd," we have enough privacy to enjoy bird song and creek song and live close to nature and to God.

I wanted a haven of peace and privacy and now we have it. Our place is like Gatlinburg without the tourists.

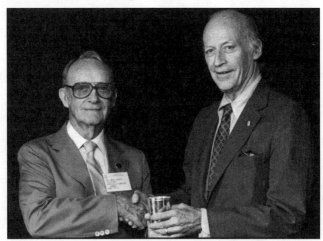

Kentucky Bankers Convention. Dr. Mack Roberts receiving community service award.

Onward

For age is opportunity no less
Than youth itself, though in another dress,
And as the evening twilight fades away,
The sky is filled with stars invisible by day.
–Henry Wadsworth Longfellow

Sometimes, as they say, we are too close to the forest to see the trees.

Reviewing our lives it is difficult to realize the years have passed so quickly. We have worked hard. We have had more than our share of good health, fun, globetrotting, romance and friendships. In addition we have known happiness and contentment. God has blessed us wonderfully.

"Memory," says Valadimir Nabokov, "is the only real estate." Our life had its emotional milestones. In a recent conversation with a friend, I mentioned that one of life's greatest experiences is becoming a parent. She agreed, then added, "Falling in love is pretty good, too!" Exactly! Great, also, was our joy in becoming grandparents and great-grandparents.

However, for me, life's ultimate experience is the new birth—my spiritual birth. Perhaps I should count my age from that time. I would be only sixty-four years old!

Believe it or not, old age has its advantages! Less is expected of us. We have fewer responsibilities and more leisure, supposedly.

The doctor continues to receive cards and letters from

patients. Some letters are from people with little education, but neither misspelled words nor twisted syntax can disguise their sincerity, love, thanks and appreciation.

The Bard of Avon stated that "the evil that men do lives after them; the good is oft interred with their bones." I should hope that Mr. Shakespeare is wrong on that score, that the good continues to live as surely as the evil.

Dr. Roberts has given his body as "a living sacrifice" (Romans 12:1) to humanity. In Wayne County he is a beloved physician.

I have been schooled in the tradition that being a wife and mother is a woman's highest calling. I found great fulfillment in my chosen role.

The doctor's mantle falls upon our grandson, Mark Looney, M.D., and who knows how many other descendants who will follow him in his profession. We are convinced that Mark will "do Granddaddy proud."

Mack and I, by the grace of God, have lived beyond the biblical three score years and ten.

A new millennium is upon us. Looking into the future of the United States, I, and even my optimistic husband, take a pessimistic view. I hope we are wrong.

Though more people are being educated, oftentimes their learning yields poor results. I find it alarming that the American murder rate is the highest in the world.

Something is terribly wrong.

Our advice to you, our dear descendants, is to profit from what older, experienced people have to say. Take advantage of those learning experiences of your ancestors. A Chinese proverb says, "To know the road ahead, ask those coming back."

Work is honorable. "An idle brain is the devil's workshop" is a true saying.

Beware of greed and materialism.

Life is too short and death is too certain to live in defiance of our God.

The accurate fulfillment of prophecy provides an overwhelming argument for the integrity, authenticity and inspiration of the Bible.

Make Christ the center of your life. Be discerning in your use of the television or computer. Spend time alone. There is a time for every thing, says the preacher in Ecclesiastes, "a time to speak and a time to keep silent." God is not found in the whirlwind of society. Set your mind on things alove. Serve the Lord with all your heart and soul. Heaven awaits the faithful.

In the evening of life, as in the fourth season, the days grow shorter. Maxwell Anderson says in "September Song,"

> *Oh, it's a long, long time*
> *From May to December*
> *But the days grow short*
> *When you reach September ....*
>
> *Oh, the days dwindle down*
> *To a precious few*
> *September, November*
> *And these precious days*
> *I'll spend with you.*

No road is so straight that it never takes a turn. My husband and I have an awareness that we, too, shall "sleep with the fathers," unless Jesus comes first. Confident of God's mercy, I welcome the afterlife. My main regret is the termination of our fifty-nine-year marriage bond at death, though I am sure God will have something better for us in the hereafter.

When I mentioned my anxiety to Mack, ever the comforter, he said, "Don't worry, Little One, we'll get together some way—and I want the first date."

Granted!

All of this and heaven, too!

All of this and heaven, too!

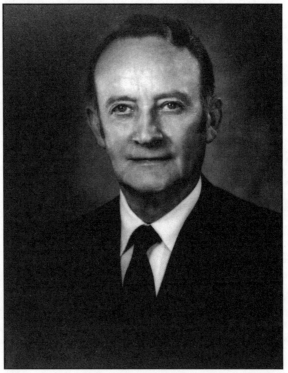

Mack Roberts, M.D.

Afterword

Since the completion of this book I have known the joy of a dream fulfilled. I have also suffered a terrible loss that I will feel for as long as I live.

In 1999, I submitted my manuscript *House Calls: Memoirs of Life with a Kentucky Doctor* to the Jesse Stuart Foundation. Probably with an awareness of our ages, Dr. James M. Gifford, the Foundation's Executive Director, graciously had the book in print in October 2000.

My husband and I were interviewed by a number of journalists; book reviews appeared in the Monticello, Kentucky *Wayne County Outlook*, the Somerset *Commonwealth Journal*, and the Sunday *Lexington Herald Leader*.

I am grateful that my husband, who coauthored several chapters, was able to enjoy the many book signings we attended: the Kentucky Authors Book Fair in Louisville, the annual Kentucky Book Fair in Frankfort, three signings at the Wayne County Bicentennial Celebration, and signings at the Monticello Banking Company in both Monticello and Somerset and at the Bank of Clinton County in Albany.

We were surprised and happy that so many friends were eager to get the book. Many relatives and friends attended the out-of-town sessions. Visiting with them was a highlight of those occasions. It did not surprise me that many buyers were more interested in getting Mack's autograph than mine. We especially enjoyed the Kentucky Book Fair in Frankfort, where our daughters Helen and Ann accompanied us. On the evening before the fair, Dr. Gifford took us to dinner, along with some of his co-workers and my former writing teacher Billy Clark and his lovely wife Ruth. What a memorable evening!

The next day both Dr. Roberts and I wore flowers in our lapels. Thousands of people attended the fair. We were surprised to see our friend Dr. Jim Taylor, president of Cumberland College, as well as former Wayne Countians. Our book attracted members of two groups, those associated with the medical profession, and the elderly, who related to the life style portrayed. Our lunch was provided, and we enjoyed a happy, successful, unforgettable day.

Following the book's publication, Mack and I were made Grand Marshals of the Christmas Parade in Monticello. He had been Grand Marshal two or three times previously.

Our book soon became available at Joseph-Beth Booksellers in Lexington, Davis-Kidd in Nashville, on the Internet, and from the Jesse Stuart Foundation, the Wayne County Library, the Monticello Banking Company at Monticello and Somerset, the Bank of Clinton County, and directly from me. I remember mailing out seventeen books in one day, and I sold hundreds of copies to people seeking Christmas gifts. We were overwhelmed at the response.

In retrospect, I have one regret about writing this book. I did not ask our three beloved daughters to contribute, simply because I wished to surprise them with the completed book as a gift. That was a great mistake. Their love and adoration of their father should have been shared; they worshiped him. He thought they were the greatest.

The main reason for writing the book was for our descendants to know Mack Roberts. The response of our great-grandson Tyler Swafford made the entire effort worthwhile. When I received the first shipment of books I immediately mailed one to each of our daughters and grandchildren. Tara Swafford, our oldest granddaughter, called the day she received it to express her thanks and appreciation. She said she had hardly seen the book because her sons—our great grandsons Tyler (age 5) and Thomas (age two)—had possessed the book, trying to identify the pictures. Then Tyler got on the phone. "Ma-mommy, did you write all those words? Where did you do it? Did you put the pictures in?"

At Thanksgiving, which we spent in Nashville, Tennessee, with Tyler's family, I took a book to each great-grandson. When I gave the book to Tyler I urged him to take good care of it, for I wanted him to keep it for *his* children. He handled the book carefully and carried it around thoughtfully. Then he asked, "How will they know who this guy is?"

"That is the reason I wrote the book—so they can read about granddaddy—and try to be like him," I said.

The next day we returned to Tyler's home. He met us at the door carrying the book. When we left, he still carried the book.

At our Christmas celebration, Tyler asked, "Ma-mommy, did your hand get tired writing that book?" A kindergartner learning to write, he must have thought it a very difficult task. Indeed, the book became a valuable keepsake for the entire family.

Completing the book was a major accomplishment in my life. I have found privacy a necessity for writing, and that was almost impossible because of the near-public nature of our home during the years when Mack was practicing medicine. Thus I was not able to write for the first seventy years of my life.

Yes, I could write a sequel. I have much more to say. I experienced true joy in reliving our lives.

Mack was my greatest encouragement. A friend told me that Mack said, "Alma did a wonderful job."

A candle burns itself out by giving light.

On March 5, 2001, Dr. Mack Roberts passed from this life at St. Joseph Hospital in Lexington, Kentucky, at age 97.

For two or three months he had experienced some angina. The pain was usually alleviated by a nitroglycerin tablet. He continued to make his daily morning trips to his office at the Monticello Banking Company. A couple of times he saw a cardiologist, who ran tests, prescribed medication, and scheduled a return appointment in June.

The angina spells were often brought on by minor exertion, such as putting his coat on. Most of his trouble occurred at night. Sometimes he would take as many as six nitroglycerine tablets during the early morning hours.

On February 22, his pain persisted after taking many of the pills. I gave him an aspirin and we took him to Wayne County Hospital, where the doctor recommended that he see a cardiologist in Lexington. Mack was transported by helicopter, but his sense of humor was unfailing; he asked the crew if they had plenty of gas. He jested again in Intensive Care when his doctor stated that a study had revealed that heart patients delivered by helicopter seemed to have profited from the vibration. Mack responded, "Do you know where I might find a good second-hand helicopter?"

On the next day Mack underwent a heart catheterization with the hope that stents could be inserted to keep the arteries open. The attempt was not successful, however, because of the extent of the blockage. The surgeon explained that two of the main arteries to the heart were completely blocked and the third was 95% blocked. Mack declined the option of surgery, and indeed even the surgeon hardly advised it in view of my husband's age.

Mack appeared completely undaunted by what was going on. Our daughters arrived, two from out of state, and we all remained with "Daddy" for thirteen days. He appeared to *enjoy* his hospital stay with the company of family and the many friends who came, called, and sent flowers and cards.

Mack's niece Rona Roberts, who lives in Lexington, visited daily, bringing flowers, reading material, and love.

The nurses loved Mack and vice versa. Indeed, the staff at St. Joseph's Hospital treated us like family.

Our spirits were lifted when the doctors began to discuss moving him somewhere for therapy, possibly in Lexington. Mack and I wanted to be at our home hospital, so I called Dr. Sherrill Roberts, our physician in Monticello. "Of course," he said, "we will be glad to admit him, but we might have to increase our security to keep all his former patients from swarming him."

Mack was able to talk by telephone with our grandson, Dr. Mark Looney, who was in Lima, Peru, studying tropical diseases. He also spoke with his sister Joyce from Ohio almost daily. He ate well and never showed anxiety though he continued to experience, I am sure, episodes of excruciating pain.

Helen, Ann, and Marilyn took turns spending nights with their father.

One weekend, Tara, Tyler, and Thomas visited. Aimee, our other granddaughter, and her youth minister husband Rob came also, as did Mack Drake, our Monticello grandson, and his father Rick. Tyler and Thomas sang and prayed for Granddaddy repeatedly. He enjoyed all of his company.

On March 5 nitroglycerine pills and morphine failed to reverse the heart problem and Mack Roberts, beloved husband and father, passed peacefully and courageously into eternity.

When Tyler learned of his grandfather's death, he again began to carry "the book." Six weeks later when he visited his grandparents, he took his book.

On March 7 I stood for twelve hours receiving callers at the funeral home, where both men and women shed tears. Everyone had a memorable tale to tell. "He *borned* me." "He delivered all fourteen of us." I was moved by their understanding and love. Our local hospital administrator said the nurses had heard Dr. Roberts might come to their hospital and they were already planning to decorate his room with flowers and balloons.

Upon the death of his friends, Dr. Roberts had always preferred to give Gideon Bibles; hundreds were given in his honor.

Thanks to Kentucky State Senator David Williams and our local Representative Ken Upchurch, our State Legislature adjourned a half day in Mack's honor. The accomplishments of Dr. Mack Roberts were noted in Washington, D.C., when Congressman Harold Rogers entered a tribute into the *Congressional Record* on March 7, 2001.

Elk Spring Valley Baptist Church could not accommodate all the mourners. The current pastor there, a former pastor, and our son-in-law Bill Looney all spoke eloquently of Mack's dedication to the Lord and his fellow man. Burial was in the Elk Spring Cemetery.

He gave us his love of life.

He gave us his life of love.

Our grandsons Tyler and Thomas continue to sing "How Great Thou Art," their grandfather's favorite song. They pray that Granddaddy's having a good time in heaven. They also sense my aloneness and include me in their prayers.

We have been overwhelmed by the love and honor shown. Tales continued to surface of Mack's devotion to his profession, and of his wit.

A former patient from Parmleysville told Marilyn, "There was no one in the world I would rather see coming to see me when I was sick than Doc Roberts. I can't tell you how many times he came out there to us." He repeated his last statement. She asked, "How did he get there?" "He walked. He would cross a branch, then go up a hill about half a mile, then cross a swinging bridge over the river, and then on a piece." Of course, Dr. Roberts had driven his Jeep to the end of the road.

In the same discussion a woman in her forties said, "They said Doc tried to buy me when I was born."

Another person added, "Our three-year-old girl idolized Dr. Roberts. During an office visit she invited him to go home with her to watch Tarzan on television. Dr. Roberts said, 'Why don't you go home with me and we'll ride ponies?' 'Oh no.' she said, 'Then we'd miss Tarzan.'"

While I visited with a friend in the hospital two ladies present discussed Dr. Roberts and his work. One remarked that he had delivered a new baby for a large family. The family asked the doctor to name the baby. "Enough," he suggested.

The pain I feel has brought me closer to God. He has not failed me, and I live on for whatever purpose God has for me.

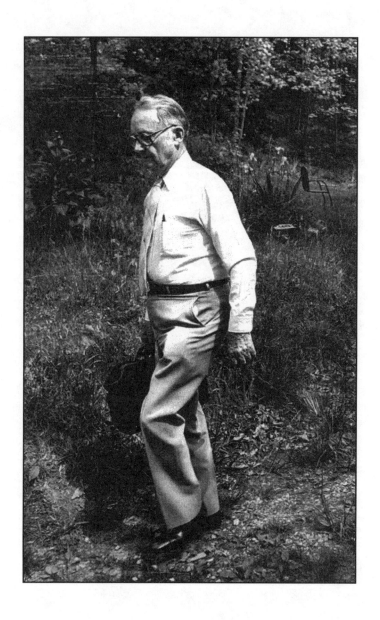

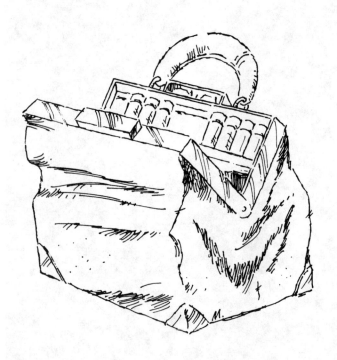